NUTRITION AND DIET RESEARCH PROGRESS

CONTEMPORARY ISSUES IN CHILDHOOD MALNUTRITION

NUTRITION AND DIET RESEARCH PROGRESS

Additional books and e-books in this series can be found on Nova's website under the Series tab.

NUTRITION AND DIET RESEARCH PROGRESS

CONTEMPORARY ISSUES IN CHILDHOOD MALNUTRITION

JYOTI RATAN GHOSH, PHD
AND
KAUSHIK BOSE, PHD
EDITORS

nova
Medicine & Health
New York

Library of Congress Cataloging-in-Publication Data

Names: Ghosh, Jyoti Ratan, editor. | Bose, Kaushik, 1962- editor.
Title: Contemporary issues in childhood malnutrition / [edited by Jyoti Ratan Ghosh and Kaushik Bose].
Description: New York : Nova Science Publishers, [2019] | Series: Nutrition and diet research progress | Includes bibliographical references and index.
Identifiers: LCCN 2020000175 (print) | LCCN 2020000176 (ebook) | ISBN 9781536173482 (hardcover) | ISBN 9781536173499 (adobe pdf)
Subjects: LCSH: Malnutrition in children. | Malnutrition in children--Case studies. | Children--Health and hygiene.
Classification: LCC RJ399.M26 .C667 2019 (print) | LCC RJ399.M26 (ebook) | DDC 362.1963/9--dc23
LC record available at https://lccn.loc.gov/2020000175
LC ebook record available at https://lccn.loc.gov/2020000176

Published by Nova Science Publishers, Inc. † New York

CONTENTS

FOREWORD

It is my great pleasure to introduce a new volume edited by Professor Kaushik Bose and Dr. Jyoti Ratan Ghosh from two universities of West Bengal, India.

It is the 6th volume edited by Professor Bose and his colleagues. The previous ones covered research topics on various aspects of thinness and obesity as the two ends of the distribution of growth parameters in children and two main evils of modern society widespread all over the world.

The new volume deals with the current aspects of childhood malnutrition, which is the continuation of the same research direction that was followed in the previous publications.

The problem of malnutrition as well as the problem of obesity is faced by many countries now, and the discussion of the studies concentrating on this issue is very timely and important.

Of course the volume does not cover all possible aspects of this complicated problem. However it highlights many of those. Among them, malnutrition and infection, malnutrition and immunization, socioeconomic and gender impacts on malnutrition, mother's nutritional status and early childhood development, etc. Some examples of undernourishment of children and adolescents in different Indian populations and how it is influencing their physical development are also given in the book.

The first entry in the volume needs special discussion. It is a paper written by the famous auxologists Michael Hermanussen, Barry Bogin and Christiane Scheffler who claim that the most important characteristic of human physical status – stature – is more influenced by social than nutritional stimuli. This is the hypothesis of so called "communal effect on growth", which presents a highly topical issue in the latest auxological and medical literature.

Such is the circle of problems discussed in the book.

I am sure that this new publication on malnutrition will be of great interest to many specialists in different fields – anthropology, pediatrics, health care, sports science, among others, as well as to the general public, to all those who are interested in children's growth and development.

In conclusion I would like to congratulate the editors with this serious undertaking and wish them to publish more new volumes in continuation of this research series dedicated to the important issues of public health care.

Elena Godina, PhD, DSci
Professor of Anatomy and Biological Anthropology
Leading Researcher, Head of Auxology Department
Institute and Museum of Anthropology,
Lomonosov Moscow State University;
Head of the Anatomy and Anthropology Department,
Russian University of Physical Education, Sports, Youth and Tourism;
Editor "VestnikMoskovskogoUniversiteta. Series XXIII.Antropologia"
Executive Editor "Journal of Physiological Anthropology and Applied Human Sciences"

PREFACE

The world is undergoing a rapid epidemiological and nutritional transition characterized by persistent nutritional deficiencies, as evidenced by the prevalence of stunting, anemia, and iron and zinc deficiencies. Concomitantly, there is a progressive rise in the prevalence of obesity.Malnutrition is one of the most important grounds for improper physical and mental development of children. The problem of low or excessive body weight concerns countries with different levels of socio-economic development. This is a medical, social, and economic issue.

Every country in the world is affected by one or more forms of malnutrition. Combating malnutrition in all its forms is one of the greatest global health challenges. Infants, children and adolescents are at particular risk of malnutrition. In children, malnutrition has particularly significant health consequences during both early development and adulthood. Malnutrition endangers children's survival, health, growth and development, slows national progress towards the developmental goals and thus diminishes the strength and capacity of nation. The developmental, economic, social, and medical impacts of the global burden of malnutrition are serious and lasting, for individuals and their families, for communities and for countries.

Nutrition research can be aimed at identifying the various social, cultural, political, and economic factors of nutrition in order to fully understand the underlying causes of malnutrition. Nevertheless, exploring the issues of food security, dietary diversity, and infant-feeding practices can provide a comprehensive understanding of a population's nutritional status.

In view of the above, this book is devoted to the issues in childhood malnutrition.Though, it is not possible to cover all aspectes of childhood malnutrition in one book, we attempt to contribute our best effort to address the issue.

In the first chapter, Hermanussen et al. discussed how stature signals social rather than nutritional status in human. It was also observed that the differences in body height between different classes are neither caused by differences in nutrition nor by differences in health.

In the next chapter Karim et al. report about gender inequalities in nutrition among under five children in rural areas of Rajshahi district, Bangladesh. The authors report that boys had more favourable nutritional status compared with girls. The study also reveals that the inferior socio-cultural position of women in the studied population.

Next, Roy and Senhave attracted our attention on the issue of polio immunization and malnutrition. The chapter presents an overview on studies that clearly depicted that malnourished children are suffering the ineffectiveness of polio vaccine.

The fourth chapter by Dutta and Sengupta highlighted on under nutrition among the adolescent Ahomchildren of upper Assam. The study shows that Ahom children are facing a risk of underweight as the prevalence of underweight is than stunting and thinness.

Mahalanabis and Sen in the fifth chapter of this book highlights on the relevance of 'thin-fat' phenotype. Moreover, the authors also developed and validated new improved tools to measure adiposity in infants and young children suitable for South Asia.

In the next chapter, Pruszkowska-Przybylskashows the influences of environmental and genetic factors on body mass and proportion among individuals on the progressive stages of ontogenesis in Poland. The paper also highlighted on malnutrition and epigenetics.

Bharati et al. in the seventh chapterdepicts the prevalence of overweight and obesity among 6-10 year children and investigates the probable risk factors of childhood obesity.The authors show that the children of private schools are more obese than public schools. The study also shows that durations of television watching, games, junk food, family history and morbidityare the risk factors for increasingchildhood obesity.

The eighth chapter by Lipoeto and Helmizar discuss on the relationship between socio-economic statuses with nutritional status among first grade school children of Padang, Indonesia. The study also reveals that the growth of children in achieving optimal growth potential is the result of adequate nutritional needs.

The next chapter on the nutritional status of tribal children under five years of age in ITDA Paderu Division of Andhra Pradesh by Sreegiri and Nayak shows that prevalence of stunting, underweight and wasting is 51%, 49.2%and 32.2%, respectively. The study also highlighted that the feeding practices in the early infancy are satisfactory, butin the late infancy and early childhood, there is deficiency in the frequency and adequacy of the feeds leading to wasting andstunting.

Ghosh et al. reported about the factors affecting thinness among school children of PurbaMedinipur, West Bengal and found that the prevalence of thinness was lower among boys compared to girls. The study also shows that parents education, fathers occupation, sanitation, number of living room and illness were significantly associated with thinness among them.

The study on health status of the rural children of Purulia, West Bengal, India by Ghosh and Chatterjeeshows poor health status of the children irrespective of economic status. The study shows that lack of diet related knowledge of the parents is the primary cause for theirpoor health status.

In chapter twelve Ghosh and Bose discuss about the interrelationship between malnutrition and childhood infections. The study reports that malnutrition as a result of disordered nutrient assimilation increase susceptibility to infections in children through impaired immunity.

We sincerely acknowledge all contributing authors for their valuable contribution, because their expertise and insights will be very helpful to the interested readers as well as researchers working on childhood malnutrition. The theme and the content of the book may also be of interest to a number of academic disciplines including biological anthropology, publichealth, epidemiology, paediatrics, nutrition, primary health care and other allied fields.

The authors also express their sincere thanks to NOVA Science Publishers, New York, U.S.A. for their support and kind cooperation, without which the publication of this book would not been possible.

Editors
Dr. Jyoti Ratan Ghosh
Prof. Kaushik Bose

In: Contemporary Issues in Childhood … ISBN: 978-1-53617-348-2
Editors: J. Ratan Ghosh and K. Bose

Chapter 1

STATURE SIGNALS SOCIAL RATHER THAN NUTRITIONAL STATUS

Michael Hermanussen[1,*], Barry Bogin[2,†] and Christiane Scheffler[3,‡]
[1]Eckernförde - Altenhof, Germany
[2]Loughborough University, School of Sport, Exercise and Health Sciences, UK
[3]University of Potsdam, Institute of Biochemistry and Biology, Human Biology, Potsdam, Germany

ABSTRACT

When human biologists, sociologists, psychologists, economists, and medical professionals consider basic social interaction patterns, it is often forgotten that people are social mammals. Competition for resources and struggle for reproductive success are universal and require adaptation strategies to the given physical and social environment. Like other social mammals, people also join together in groups, experience group

* Corresponding Author's Email: michael.hermanussen@gmail.com.
† Corresponding Author's Email: b.a.bogin@lboro.ac.uk.
‡ Corresponding Author's Email: christiane.scheffler@uni-potsdam.de.

membership, are superior or dominant over some people, "at eye level" with other group members, but are also excluded or dominated by some and are required to "pull their heads in" - "make themselves small" - in order to survive the competition with the greatest possible success.

It has long been known that body height and mass have signaling functions among social mammals (Cinnirella and Winter 2009). This also applies for humans. Humans are able to perceive physical size as a signal of social dominance. The greater influence of perceived taller humans in a negotiation task has been described by Huang et al. (Huang et al. 2002). Taller men are perceived as more competent and authoritative (e.g., Young and French 1996; Judge and Cable 2004; Cinnirella and Winter 2009). Also, children watching interactions between other people recognize cues that predict dominance such as differences in physical size and number of people forming an alliance (Lourenco et al. 2016).

Dominance and Body Height

Recent studies in wild Kalahari meerkats (*Suricata suricatta*) suggested that social dominance itself can be a strong growth impulse. Meerkats that, "…acquire dominant status, show a secondary period of accelerated growth whose magnitude increases if the difference between their own weight and that of the heaviest subordinate of the same sex in their group is small" (Huchard et al. 2016). It is the relative, not the absolute size that serves as the signal for. "…individuals (to) adjust their growth to the size of their closest competitor". If, for example, the growth of individual animals that are low in the group hierarchy is stimulated beyond the usual level by targeted supplementary feeding, hierarchically higher group members may feel threatened. This threat can increase the growth rate. Meerkats adapt individual growth rates competitively to social conditions. They grow "strategically". Huchard et al. showed that the abolition of reproductive suppression and the reorientation of life history strategies with the acquisition of a dominant position is accompanied by corresponding hormonal changes, with higher estradiol and progesterone levels in females and higher cortisol levels in both sexes. Also, in other social species subordination leads to inhibition of growth and dominance to stimulation of growth.

Sapolsky and Spencer (1997) investigated the relationship between social status and IGF-1 (Insulin-like Growth Factor 1) in baboons and observed that social subordination was associated with suppression of IGF-1 concentration. Bartos and colleagues (1998) showed in *Pudus*, a South American deer species, that from September to November (the second part of the antler growth period), the IGF-1 levels of dominant males were significantly higher than those of subordinate males.

Body height and IGF-1 are related. But relations between social status and IGF-1 are hardly described in humans. Kumari and Mitarbeiter (2008) investigated the association between social position, measured by paternal or own occupational class, and IGF-1. Low IGF-1 values were associated with lower social position. The association was valid for adults and was independent of the social position at birth.

The small number of endocrinological studies in individuals does not immediately reveal whether the principles of strategic growth adjustments also apply to humans, as already suggested by Huchard et al. (2016). However, extensive historical data suggests that strategic growth also plays a role in humans.

In contrast to meerkats who do not stop growing at the beginning of the reproductive age, humans are usually fully grown at a time when they start to achieve leading positions in society. As strategic adjustments of growth and body height cannot take place after adolescence, short adults who occupy important positions thus, often tend to underline their social role by particularly behavior - everyone is familiar with the "little Napoleon" or "short man" complex.

In human adolescents, even the prospect of a later dominant social position seems to stimulate growth. Kings and members of the aristocracy have always grown taller than the ordinary people. Height measurements of High Carls School students from the late 18th century show that young aristocrats grew significantly taller than their non-aristocratic schoolmates – irrespective of diet, health and general living conditions (Hartmann 1970). This is an interesting story.

Between 1763 and 1767, the Duke Carl Eugen of Württemberg had a hunting lodge built near Stuttgart. His adjutant, Colonel von Seeger, suggested that he set up a school for children of military soldiers in the adjoining buildings of the palace. This soon developed into a military academy, the so-called Hohe Carlsschule, where the young people were subjected to a strict but excellent education under the eyes of the sovereign. Many officers, civil servants and people from the state now sent their sons to this institution which gradually transformed into an elite educational institution. Snobbery and other discriminatory behavior based on social differences were not tolerated. School lessons lasted eight hours a day, including physical exercises and drill hours. The boys wore uniforms, were subject to military ceremonial, and lived in military barracks.

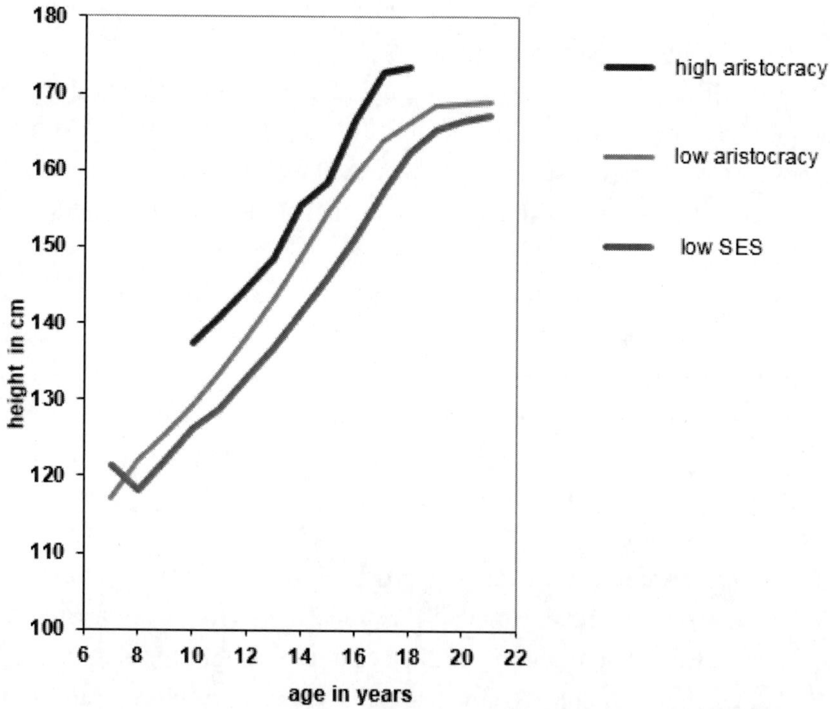

Figure 1. Body height of Carlsschule students from high aristocracy, lower aristocracy and lower social classes (low SES). The young aristocrats were on average 10cm taller than youths from the lower social classes. The young people only differed in their future prospects, rather expecting an aristocratic, or a more subordinate life style.

In the beginning there were no holidays at all, later only very short ones, so that teachers and pupils practically constantly lived together. The body size of the pupils was regularly measured and there are large sets of data on more than 1000 boys, some of which were measured over many years at very regular intervals (Hartmann 1970).

Figure 1 shows body height of Carlsschule students from high aristocracy, low aristocracy and lower social classes. The young aristocrats were on average 10cm taller than youths from the lower social classes, regardless of equal living conditions of all the boys and even the traumatic separation from their parents' lifestyle. These young people only differed in their future prospects: some expected an aristocratic, i.e., dominant social life, the others subordination.

Social differences in body height have long been known. Schlesinger explicitly wrote in 1925 (Schlesinger 1925):

> "The length curves of grammar school students and upper secondary school students are always several centimeters higher than those of elementary school students [did not attemd grammar or secondary school]. The lowest curve is that of the children from the auxiliary school, most of whom originated from the lower proletariat. The growth advantage of the well-developed, well-situated boys from the grammar schools over their less well-off peers from the elementary school equals at least a one year's growth rate in length, later in childhood and compared with less well-developed children, their growth rate may double or even exceed 2-3 years' growth rates. The difference in growth rate is not only great, it is also extraordinarily regular. The average lengths of groups of children of the same age and of the same developmental level allow a reliable classification of the social composition of those groups. In terms of weight gain, these differences are far from being so great and regular. Before puberty the differences correspond to half or three quarters of an annual amount of growth".

These social class differences could not be explained by the amount or quality of food eaten by the children. Numerous publications before, during and after the First World War underline that differences in body height between different classes are neither caused by differences in nutrition nor by differences in health (Hermanussen et al. 2018a,b).

Community and Body Height

Eveleth and Tanner (1990) wrote "Human differ in size". Children of tall parents tend to grow taller than children of short parents. There are tall populations – Dutch men have an average height of 184 cm and are currently considered the tallest (Fredriks et al. 2000) – and there are short populations, such as people from Guatemala or Indonesia. Since a long time, these observations gave rise to speculations about the genetics of body height. The literature is still full of estimates claiming that some 60% to 80% of body height variation is supposed to be genetic. This is not true. Around 1865 Dutch recruits were on average 163cm tall; i.e., shorter than modern Indonesians. At present, modern Indonesian adolescents grow similar to Hamburg Latin school students in 1879 (Kotelmann 1879). The amazing increments in body height of Europeans started at the beginning of the 20th century. The NCD Risk Factor Collaboration (NCD-Risk 2016) described changes in average body height of up to plus 20cm within populations during the last hundred years. During the past century several very short national groups became very tall and some of the tallest in the past are today relatively short. People of European origin in the United States of America were the tallest in world in the year 1900 but today rank 38th of the 201 nations in the NCD-Risk database. The relatively slow generational sequence of human societies, with comparatively small number of descendants and thus relatively little change in the genome of a society, suggests that the body height trends in the course of only four to five generations can hardly be explained by genetics. Using genome-wide association study (GWAS), Tyrrell et al. (2016) described that the 396 genetic variants studied by them explained only 12.3% of the variance in adult size. In contrast to the high variability of body height between populations, the variability of body height within populations appears rather small. More than 10 years ago, Christakis and Fowler (2007) described the spread of obesity in social networks and highlighted the similarity in weight among people who know each other: you are always as fat as your friends. This also applies to body height. Studies of Swiss and Norwegian military conscripts showed that height is related within geographically neighboring districts (Bents et al. 2017, 2018). People whose places of residence are close to each other are more similar in height than people who do not or rarely meet. We call this "community effect in body height" (Assmann and Hermanussen 2013). The community effect in body height describes the "effect of social interaction within a group, on growth and body height of its members". The physiology underlying this phenomenon is unknown, but the corresponding demographic statistics are impressive. Figure 2 shows the distribution of body height of Swiss (Schaffhausen) conscripts of the late 19th and late 20th century. Average height of this population has increased by almost 15cm: whereas 100 years ago, nobody was tall – only single individuals grew taller than 182cm – today, hardly anybody stays below 165cm, i.e., the median male size 100 years ago (Hermanussen 2013).

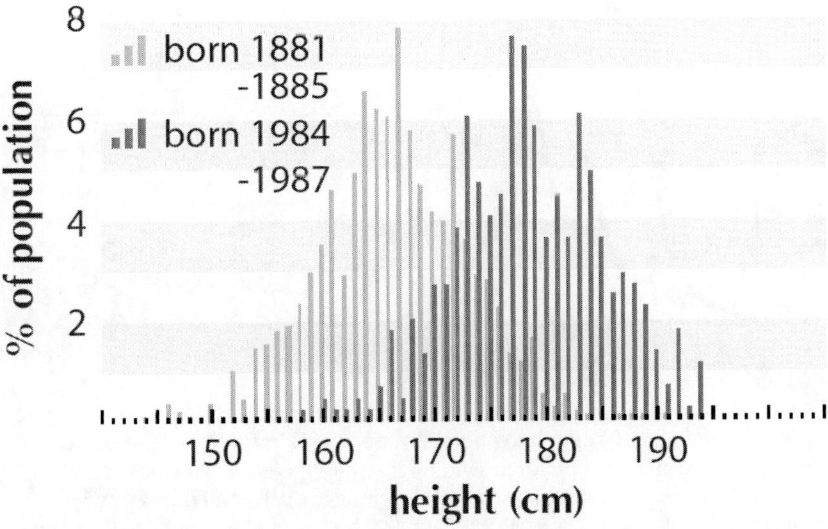

Figure 2. Distribution of body height of Swiss (Schaffhausen) conscripts of the late 19th and late 20th century. Average height of this population has increased by almost 15cm (Hermanussen 2013, reprinted with kind permission of Schweizerbart).

Body height adjustments are not necessarily slow phenomena that take place during long historical periods. Children of migrants and adolescents with lower social status adjust in height to the average body height of their new reference population already within the first generation (Bogin et al. 2018). Figure 3 shows the "community effect in body height" among children of Guatemalan parents who lived in Guatemala and children who migrated to the USA. Migrant children had grown one and a half to two standard deviations (about 8-12cm depending on age) taller than their nephews and cousins who had stayed in Guatemala.

Spier (1929) described the adaptation of migrant body height to height of the new peer-group some 90 years ago in Japanese people who grew up in the USA.

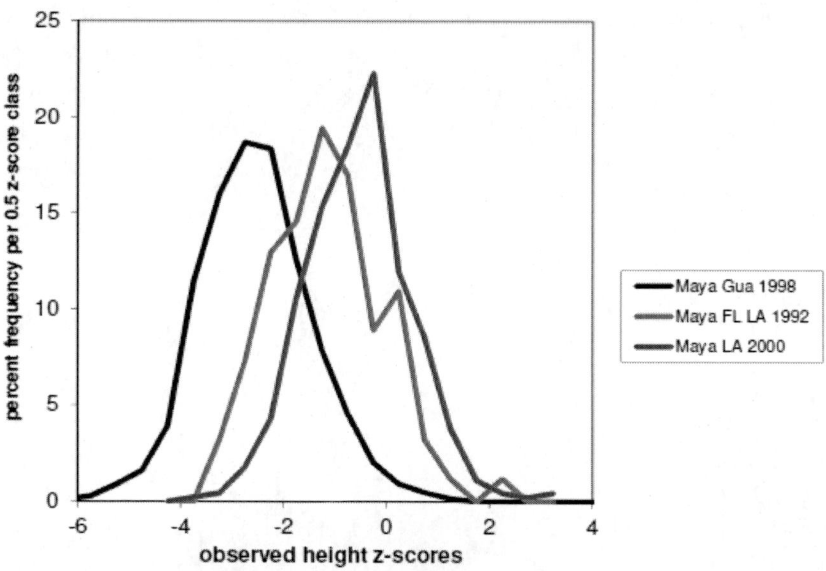

Figure 3. "Community effect in body height" among children of Guatemalan parents who lived in Guatemala and children who migrated to the USA. Height is given in height standard deviation (z-) scores referred to modern WHO references. Migrant children (Maya FL LA 1992 and Maya LA 2000) had grown one and a half to two standard deviations (about 8-12cm depending on age) taller than their nephews and cousins who had stayed in Guatemala (Maya Gua 1998). 'Maya FL La 1992' and 'Maya La 2000' refer to groups of ethnically Maya children, ages 5-12 years old, measured in Florida or Los Angeles, California in the years 1992 and 2000 (Bogin et al. 2018).

Spier found no explanation for this phenomenon, in particular, no evidence of dietary influence.

Body Height and Nutrition

Apart of the belief in genetic influences, nutrition has also been assigned an important role in the regulation of growth. Lartey (2015) writes: "There is increasing agreement among the nutrition community about the use of length/height-for-age as the indicator to monitor the long-term impact of chronic nutritional deficiencies".

Lartey calls stunting (stunting is defined as growth and developmental disorders experienced by children through poor nutrition, repeated infections and inadequate psychosocial stimulation) an "indicator of linear growth failure", with "both long- and short-term consequences affecting growth and development and adult work potential". Prendergast and Humphrey (2014) identified a "stunting syndrome" in developing countries.

And Black et al. (2013) estimated that 165 million children under the age of 5 are chronically malnourished.

Children with a z-score value for body height below -2, are by definition regarded as "stunted", i.e., malnourished. Z-score values are statistical measures. They indicate the position of a measured value within its distribution using the standard deviation. If a person's body height is 2 standard deviations below the population mean, he or she has a z-score value of minus 2.

Expressed as a percentage, a z-score of -2 says that about two and a half percent of all people of the same age and sex are shorter, and 97.5% taller, than that person.

The belief in an association between "stunting" and malnutrition has existed since the early 1970s (Waterlow 1972) and the term stunting as a synonym for malnutrition in the scientific literature became widely adopted following an international Nestle workshop in 1988 (Waterlow 1988).

This was not always the case. Already at the end of the 19th century and – this makes these observations so remarkable – explicitly in view of the catastrophic nutritional situation of the German civilian population after World War I, German paediatricians wrote that "…the longitudinal growth of the child is largely independent of the extent and type of nutrition...". (Schlesinger 1919). Similar reports were made by other European paediatricians.

It is not always easy to assess the nutritional status of a child. Based on the vision that the thickness of the subcutaneous fat layer allows statements on the nutrition status, many publications have been published in recent years, but none of them found a sustainable relationship between subcutaneous fat depot and body height. Figure 4 shows our own observations on body height (z-score values according to WHO references) and triceps and subscapular skinfold thickness of healthy 1st to 6th grade schoolchildren of a rural (Soe) and an urban region (Kupang) in West Timor, Indonesia. The inhabitants of this Indonesian island can be considered genetically similar, the everyday food is still quite traditional. Only in the few urban centers, fast food packed in small plastic bags is increasingly offered.

The rural children of Soe are very short; some 50% are stunted, with body height below minus 2 standard deviations (WHO reference), i.e., below the 2.5th centile of the reference population.

The children of Kupang are on average one standard deviation taller (approx. 5 - 6cm), but the number of "stunted children" is still high. According to international definition, these children must be considered chronically malnourished. Yet, the figure lacks evidence of a relevant association between skinfold thickness and body height. Children with little subcutaneous fat are not the shortest, and children with thicker fat tissue are not the tallest, neither in Soe nor in Kupang. The variation of the body height distribution is very similar in both populations (Scheffler et al. 2019).

Recent Indian data from "stunted children" of urban Kolkata (Scheffler et al. 2018) similarly lack an association between height and nutritional status, as measured by the strength of skinfold thickness. Even the overweight children are short when referred on global references.

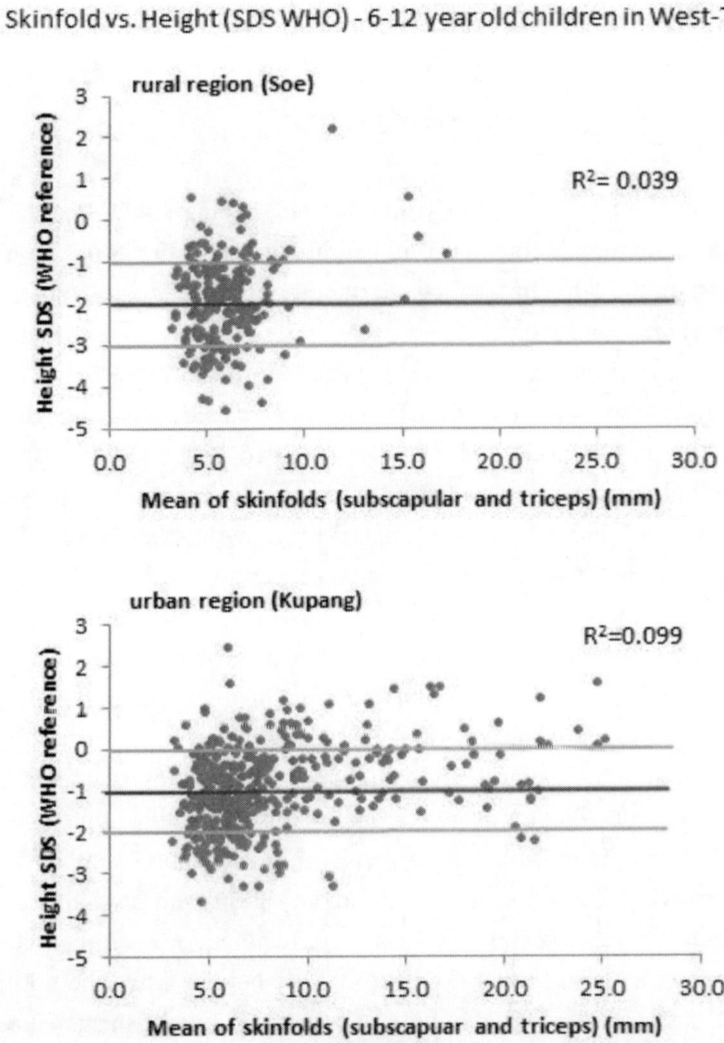

Figure 4. Body height (z-scores, WHO reference) and triceps and subscapular skinfold thickness of healthy 1st to 6th grade schoolchildren of a rural (Soe) and an urban region (Kupang) in West Timor/Indonesian. The red line indicates average z-scores. According to international definition, many children must be considered chronically malnourished, but with $R^2 = 0.04$, respectively, $R^2 = 0.1$, the figure lacks evidence of a relevant association between skinfold thickness and body height.

The Dynamics of Body Height Trends as Expressions of Social and Political Circumstances

The association between body height and social strata, the ethnic variability, and the remarkable trends in height during the last century on the one hand, and on the other hand, the lack of convincing evidence for genetic and nutritional reasons for these patterns, suggest alternative interpretations, especially in view of recent observations in social mammals.

As discussed above, social dominance itself can be a strong growth impulse in Kalahari meerkats (Huchard et al. 2016). Meerkats are able to adapt individual growth rates and grow "strategically". Subordination may lead to growth inhibition and dominance to growth stimulation. These observations are new. If we assume that such social influences on the control of growth, the capacity for competitive growth, and the "strategic" adjustment of body height are also part of human growth regulation, such assumptions are radical. They do not only put many modern, but many historical observations on growth and data on adult height in a very different light. Huchard and colleagues showed via controlled experiments that subordinate meerkats that are growth stimulated by targeted supplementary feeding start to threaten their hierarchically higher group members who respond by growing faster than usual without any additional food intake. Let us assume that like these social meerkats, also members of the human lower social strata start to "strategically" adjust in body height, when the political situation starts to promise social upgrade and a better future. In such a case, we must expect major dynamics in the body height of the upper social classes during these historic periods. In fact, this is the case.

In feudal systems where social rank is inherited, class affiliations are rigid and changes of class are rare. Such systems in fact lack dynamics in growth. Aristocrats were generally taller than the common people (Figure 1). Historic European military data show stability in body height up to the end of the 19th century. The wave of social revolutions of the first half of the 19th century was suppressed throughout Europe. Only in the Netherlands, the uprising in 1848 and 1849 led to democratic reforms. In Germany the three-class right to vote persisted until the end of the imperial era. Figure 5 illustrates the changes of height of European conscripts, with significant height trends since the mid-19th century only in the Dutch (Kenntner 1963).

After World War I, the political situation changed in most European countries, and so did growth and height. Koch wrote in 1935:

> "... even when they (adolescents) are on a starvation diet, their size ruthlessly increases until their bodies have used up their last depots. One could even speak of a "parasitic" growth in length! Even during the years of severe hunger and the years of greatest unemployment, there was no, or only a very slight decrease in the average height of schoolchildren compared to the pre-war period".

And Schlesinger wrote in 1925:

> "A completely new view on this issue was provided by Pfaundler who did not consider the short stature of the underprivileged children as the deviant, but on the contrary, rather discussed the excessive tallness of the children of the rich".

In other words, one the most famous physicians in those days, the Austrian-German pediatrician Meinhard von Pfaundler (1872 - 1947), considered the highly stimulated growth of young people from wealthy families to be pathology.

Revolutions stir up hope. Hopes of social advancement and future dominance stimulate growth, and lead to increasing height of young lower-class people.

When this increase in height is perceived as social challenge in the dominant strata, it may cause upward trends in their body height, and ultimately, may lead to a "strategic" upward spiral of body height growth of the entire population. Exactly this is found in the historic data.

Periods of democratization, but also times of political turmoil, when social equality is promised and vertical mobility and an ascent from the lower social strata becomes feasible, seem to be the motor of the exceptional body height increase observed in the European people since the end of the feudal period. The opposite also occurs as is the case for African-American women whose average adult height declined by 1.42cm in the first decade of the 21st century, while average height for European-American women increased slightly (Komlos 2010). During that decade, inequality between blacks and whites increased in many social and economic indicators (https://www.epi.org/publication/50-years-after-the-kerner-commission/).

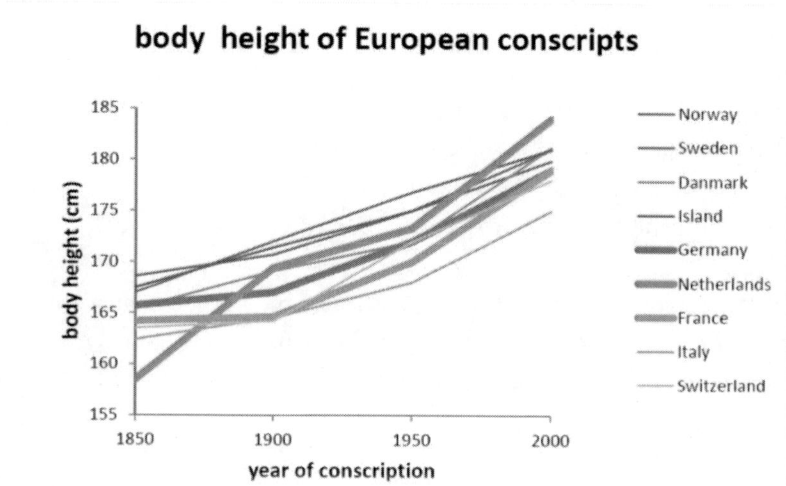

Figure 5. Body height of European conscripts, with significant height trends since the mid-19th century only in the Dutch (Kenntner 1963).

Considering this social and political mechanism, we can no longer simply explain the shortness of many Third World populations as an expression of chronic malnutrition - indeed, modern Cochrane Systematic Reviews (Visser et al. 2018) underline the insignificance of nutrition interventions in these countries, "Considering the current evidence base included, supplementary food effects are modest at best" (ibid). We understand the absence of secular height trends in these populations as an expression of persistent feelings of being inferior. South Africans named this inferiority complex by coining the term "white privilege"; be it the consequence of colonial rule, be it lack of education, or an expression of perceived patronization in the face of the global spread and dominance of Western life and moral codes.

REFERENCES

Aßmann, C., Hermanussen, M. (2013). Modeling determinants of growth: evidence for a community-based target in height? *Pediatr. Res.*Jul.; 74(1):88 - 95.

Bartos, L., Reyes, E., Schams, D., Bubenik, G., Lobos, A. (1998). Rank dependent seasonal levels of IGF-1, cortisol and reproductive hormones in male pudu (Pudu puda). *Comp. Biochem. Physiol. A Mol. Integr. Physiol.,* Jun.; 120(2):373 - 8.

Bents, D., Groth, D., Satake, T. (2018). The secular trend and network effects on height of male Japanese students from 1955 to 2015. *Anthropol. Anz.,* Jun. 11; 74(5):423 - 429.

Bents, D., Rybak, A., Groth, D. (2017). Spatial conscript body height correlation of Norwegian districts in the 19(th) century. *Anthropol. Anz.,* Apr. 1; 74(1):65 - 69.

Black, R. E., Victora, C. G., Walker, S. P., Bhutta, Z. A., Christian, P., de Onis, M., Ezzati, M., Grantham-McGregor, S., Katz, J., Martorell, R., Uauy, R. (2013). Maternal and Child Nutrition Study Group. Maternal and child undernutrition and overweight in low-income and middle-income countries. *Lancet,* Aug. 3; 382(9890):427 - 451.

Bogin, B., Hermanussen, M., Scheffler, C. (2018). As tall as my peers - similarity in body height between migrants and hosts. *Anthropol. Anz.,* Jun. 11; 74(5):365 - 376.

Cinnirella, F., Winter, J. (2009). *Size matters! Body height and labor market discrimination: a cross-European analysis.* – CESifo Working Paper Series. pp. 1 - 29.

Eveleth, P. B., Tanner, J. M. (1990). Worldwide variation in human growth. 2nd ed. *Cambridge University Press.* Cambridge.

Fredriks, A. M., Buuren, Sv., Burgmeijer, R. J. F., Meulmeester, J. F., Beuker, R. J., Brugman, E., Roede, M. J., Verloove-Vanhorick, S. P.,

Wit, J. M. (2000) Continuing positive secular growth change in the Netherlands 1955-1997. *Ped. Res.*:47:316 -323.

Hartmann, W. (1970). *Beobachtungen zur Akzeleration des Längenwachstums in der zweiten Hälfte des 18. Jahrhunderts. Carlsschule* "[Observations on the acceleration of longitudinal growth in the second half of the 18th century. "Carls School"]. Dissertation. Frankfurt.

Hermanussen, M., Bogin, B., Scheffler, C. (2018a). Stunting, starvation and refeeding: a review of forgotten 19th and early 20th century literature. *Acta Paediatr.,* Jul.; 107(7):1166 - 1176.

Hermanussen, M., Bilogub, M., Lindl, A. C., Harper, D., Mansukoski, L., Scheffler, C. (2018b). Weight and height growth of malnourished school-age children during re-feeding. Three historic studies published shortly after World War I. *Eur. J. Clin. Nutr.,* Aug. 30. doi: 10.1038/ s41430-018-0274-z.

Hermanussen, M. (ed) (2013). Studying Human Growth and Development. *Schweizerbart Science Publishers*, Stuttgart.

Huang, W., Olson, J. S., Olson, G. M. (2002). Camera angle affects dominance in video-mediated communication. In: *Proceedings of the Conference on Human Factors in Computing Systems.* Association for Computing Machinery. New York. pp. 716 - 717.

Huchard, E., English, S., Bell, M. B., Thavarajah, N., Clutton-Brock, T. (2016). Competitive growth in a cooperative mammal. *Nature,* 533 (7604): 532 - 534.

Judge, T. A., Cable, D. M. (2004). The effect of physical height on workplace success and income: preliminary test of a theoretical model. *J. Appl. Psychol.,* 89: 428 - 441.

Kenntner, G. (1963). Die Veränderungen der Körpergröße des Menschen. Eine biogeographische Untersuchung. [*The changes in human body height. A biogeographical examination*] Dissertation. Karlsruhe.

Koch, E. W. (1935). Über die Veränderung menschlichen Wachstums im ersten Drittel des 20. Jahrhunderts [*About the change in human growth in the first third of the 20th century.*] Barth. Leipzig.

Komlos, J. (2010). The recent decline in the height of African-American women. *Economics and Human Biology,* 8:58 - 66.

Kotelmann, L. (1879). Die Körperverhältnisse der Gelehrtenschüler des Johanneums in Hamburg: Ein statistischer Beitrag zur Schulhygiene.[*The body conditions of the scholarly students of the Johanneum in Hamburg: A statistical contribution to school hygiene.*] Zeitschrift des Königlichen Preussischen statistischen Bureau's. Berlin.

Kumari, M., Tabassum, F., Clark, C., Strachan, D., Stansfeld, S., Power, C. (2015). Social differences in insulin-like growth factor-1: *findings from a British birth Cohort Ann. Epidemiol.,* 2008; 18:664 - 70. Lartey A. What would it take to prevent stunted growth in children in sub-Saharan Africa? *Proc. Nutr. Soc.,* 74:449 - 53.

Lourenco, S. F., Bonny, J. W., Schwartz, B. L. (2016). Children and Adults Use Physical Size and Numerical Alliances in Third-Party Judgments of Dominance. *Front. Psychol.,* 6: 2050.

NCD Risk Factor Collaboration (NCD-RisC). (2016). A century of trends in adult human height. *Elife.* 26; 5. pii: e13410. doi: 10.7554/eLife.13410.

Prendergast, A. J., Humphrey, J. H. (2014). The stunting syndrome in developing countries. – *Paediatr. Int. Child Health,* 34 (4):250 - 265.

Sapolsky, R. M., Spencer, E. M. (1997). Insulin-like growth factor I is suppressed in socially subordinate male baboons. *Am. J. Physiol.,* 273 (4 Pt 2): R1346 - 51.

Scheffler, C., Krützfeldt, L. M., Dasgupta, P., Hermanussen, M. (2018). No association between fat tissue and height in 5019 children and adolescents, measured between 1982 and in 2011 in Kolkata/India. *Anthropol. Anz.,* 74:403 - 411.

Scheffler, C., Hermanussen, M., Bogin, B., Liana, D. S., Taolin, F., Cempaka, P. M. V. P., Irawan, M., Ibbibah, L. F., Mappapa, N. K., Payong, M. K. E., Homalessy, A. V., Takalapeta, A., Apriyanti, S., Manoeroe, M. G., Dupe, F. R., Ratri, R. R. K., Touw, S. Y., K. P. V., Murtani, B. J., Nunuhitu, R., Puspitasari, R., Riandra, I. K., Liwan, A. S., Amandari, P., Permatasari, A. A. I., Julia, M., Batubara, J., Pulungan, A.(2019). Stunting is not a synonym of malnutrition. *Eur. J. Clin. Nutr.,* May 29. doi: 10.1038/s41430-019-0439-4.

Schlesinger, E. (1925). Das Wachstum des Kindes. [The growth of the child] *Ergebnisse der inneren Medizin und Kinderheilkunde,* 28:456 - 579.

Schlesinger, E. (1919). Wachstum, Gewicht und Konstitution der Kinder und der heranwachsenden Jugend während des Krieges. [Growth, weight and constitution of children and adolescent youth during the war] *Zeitschrift für Kinderheilkunde,* 22: 80 - 123.

Spier, L. (1929). Growth of Japanese children born in America and in Japan. University of Washington Publication in Anthropology V3 No1.

Tyrrell, J., Jones, S. E., Beaumont, R., Astley, C. M., Lovell, R., Yaghootkar, H., Tuke, M., Ruth, K. S., Freathy, R. M., Hirschhorn, J. N., Wood, A. R., Murray, A., Weedon, M. N., Frayling, T. M. (2016). Height, body mass index, and socioeconomic status: mendelian randomisation study in UK Biobank. *BMJ,* Mar. 8; 352:i582.

Visser, J., McLachlan, M. H., Maayan, N., Garner, P. (2018). Community-based supplementary feeding for food insecure, vulnerable and malnourished populations - an overview of systematic reviews. *Cochrane Database Syst. Rev.,* Nov. 9; 11:CD010578.

Waterlow, J. C. (1972). Classification and definition of protein-calorie malnutrition. – *Brit. Med. J.,* 3 (5826): 566 - 569.

Waterlow, J. C. (1988). Observations on the Natural History of Stunting. – In: Waterlow, J. C. (ed.): *Linear Growth Retardation in Less Developed Countries.* Nestlé Nutrition Workshop Series 1988. Vol. 14. Nestec Ltd., Vevey/Raven Press Ltd., New York.

Young, T. J., French, L. A. (1996). Height and perceived competence of US presidents. *Perceptual and Motor Skills,* 82: 1002.

In: Contemporary Issues in Childhood … ISBN: 978-1-53617-348-2
Editors: J. Ratan Ghosh and K. Bose ©2020 Nova Science Publishers, Inc.

Chapter 2

ASSOCIATION BETWEEN CHILDREN'S NUTRITIONAL STATUS AND SOCIO-DEMOGRAPHIC FACTORS: GENDER INEQUALITY

Reazul Karim[1], MD, Masud Rana[1], MD, Abdul Wadood[2] and Golam Hossain[1,*], MD
[1]Health Research Group, Department of Statistics,
University of Rajshahi, Rajshahi, Bangladesh
[2]Deputy Chief Medical Officer, University of Rajshahi,
Rajshahi, Bangladesh

ABSTRACT

The rate of literacy and household wealth index have been increasing during last two decades, still gender inequality is a big problem in Bangladesh regarding health and nutritional status. The objective of the study was to investigate the association between children nutritional status

* Corresponding Author's Email: hossain95@yahoo.com.

and socio-demographic factors. Also, we wanted to look gender inequality in nutrition among children under five years old in the rural area of Rajshahi district, Bangladesh.

It was a cross-sectional study with a sample size of 540 children (aged 6-59 months). Data were collected from the field survey conducted from October to December 2016 in the rural areas of Rajshahi district, Bangladesh by using multistage sampling technique.

Chi-square (χ^2)-test was used to examine the associations between under five children (aged 6-59 months) nutritional status and socio-demographic factors with gender inequlity. Binary logistic regression was used to find the effects of socio-demographic on the nutritional status among the children (aged 6-59 months).

This study revealed that the prevalence of stunting children was 43.7%, among them 46.4% and 41.0% were girls and boys respectively. The binary logistic model demonstrated that fathers who spent ≥ 6 hours at home were less likely to have stunted boys than those who spent less time (AOR = 0.360, 95% CI: 0.159-0.815; p < 0.05). Boys who came from a female headed household were more likely to become stunted than their counterpart (AOR = 0.412, 95% CI: 0.173-0.983; $p < 0.05$). The mothers who didn't received antenatal care services had more chance to have stunted boys than who were received antenatal care services (AOR = 3.611, 95% CI: 1.537-8.487; p < 0.01). It was found that fathers who spent ≥ 6 hours at home were less likely to have stunted girls than those who spent less time (AOR = 0.226, 95% CI: 0.097-0.524 $p < 0.01$). Girls who came from poor households were more likely to become stunted than their counterpart (AOR = 0.437, 95% CI: 0.195-0.978; $p < 0.05$). In this study explored that short mothers (height ≤145cm) were more likely to have stunted girls than taller mothers (height >145 cm) (AOR = 0.383, 95% CI: 0.163-0.900; $p < 0.05$). Girls who had ≥6 members household were less likely to become stunted than the girls living with less than 3 members household (AOR = 0.396, 95% CI: 0.175-0.896; $p < 0.05$). The mothers who didn't receive TT injection during pregnancy had more chance to have stunted girls than who received TT injection during pregnancy (AOR = 0.529, 95% CI: 0.284-0.985; $p < 0.05$). The mothers who didn't take iron-folic supplementation during pregnancy had more chance to have stunted girls than who took iron-folic supplementation during pregnancy (AOR = 0.300, 95% CI: 0.099-0.905; $p < 0.05$). The prevalence of underweight among preschool children was 39.6%, and the prevalence of girls (40.8%) was higher than that of boys (38.5%). The model demonstrated that boys aged 6-24 months had more chance to have underweight than their counterpart (AOR = 0.503, 95% CI: 0.279-0.908; $p < 0.05$). Fathers who spent ≥6 hours at home were less likely to have underweight girls than those who spent less than ≤ 2 hours (AOR = 0.383, 95% CI: 0.159-0.922; $p < 0.05$).

Our findings show that boys had better nutritional status than that of girls. Socio-demographic and nutritional service had positive impact on nutritional status but unfortunately gender inequality still persist. An improvement of girls' health and nutritional status to a level of boys needs broad-based interventions.

Keywords: gender inequality, nutritional status, multiples logistic regression, Rajshahi district

BACKGROUND

Gender refers to the socially constructed characteristics of women and men, this includes norms, roles and relationships that exist between them (WHO, 2015). Gender inequality is the idea and situation that women and men are not equal (Wood, 2005). It means the existence of social norms and culture and even laws and rules that result in differential access to control over resources, services and opportunities based on the sex (Balgir, 2009). It arises from differences in socially constructed gender roles and refers to unequal treatment due to their gender and often it is dichotomous and hierarchical. Nutritional status is the levels of nutrients in the body which is influenced by the diet and utilization of nutrients (Bender, 2005), and it is usually measured by anthropometric measurements such as body mass index (BMI) for adults and height for age, weight for age, weight for height, and BMI percentile for children. (WHO, 2006). Nutritional status further greatly influences an individual's growth, educational attainment, productivity, reproductive success and susceptibility to disease (Marphatia, 2016). Malnutrition the extreme negative of nutritional status, is an abnormal physiological condition caused by deficiencies, excesses or imbalances in energy, protein and/or other nutrients, and resulting diet-related non-communicable diseases (WHO, 2018).

Globally 20% of child deaths are still related to malnutrition (WHO, 2017). Gender equality in nutrition remains a big problem in major parts of the world, particularly in developing countries. Improvements in nutritional equality in gender are important to achieving the Sustainable Development

Goals (SDGs), ending hunger and improving nutrition have remaineds a top priority for international development. It is closely linked to some goals of SDG such as number 2 of the SDGs (zero hunger) and number 5 (gender equality). It strives to contribute to goals by exploring the link between malnutrition and gender equality (Assembly, 2015).

Gender inequality in nutrition is strongly associated with eating, food distribution and nutritional habits that influence women and/or men nutritional status. Women and girls are the main victims of the "food discrimination," which results in chronic undernutrition and ill health (FAO, 2015). Gender inequality can be a cause as well as an effect of hunger and malnutrition. Not surprisingly, higher levels of gender inequality are associated with higher levels of undernutrition, both acute and chronic undernutrition (Mucha, 2012). Gender inequality and malnutrition through their influence and interaction with health conditions affect different aspects and dimensions of socioeconomic development (World Bank, 2006).

Although many developing countries succeeded in reducing undernutrition, most of them failed to significantly reduce the inequalities (Bredenkamp, 2014). Girls and women are exposed to all sorts of discrimination, abuse, and exploitation and often have less access to nutrition (Dey, 2008). Income controlled by women is more frequently used on food and health care for the family and especially for children (UNICEF, 2011; Smith et al. 2003). Gender inequities and dynamics are a major social determinant of health and nutrition outcomes (CSDH, 2008). Several studies have also reported that empowered mothers were able to reduce inequality in nutritional status between boys and girls (Bose, 2011). Gender inequality in nutritional status due to intra household allocation of resources has been consistently reported in several parts of South Asia (Dey and Chaudhuri, 2008; Moestue, 2008; Dancer et al. 2008). Gender inequalities in quantity and quality of food intake may contribute to under-nutrition mainly in settings where the girl child is still considered less important than the boy child (Jawaregowda, 2015). One of the reasons believed to continue food insecurity is the discrimination against women (Assan, 2013). Gender differences in nutrition argue that household power relations are closely linked to nutritional outcomes. When men had complete control over all decisions, women had significantly lower nutritional status than men (Vlassoff, 2007).

In many societies women and girls eat the remaining food after the male family members have eaten (FAO, 2015). Research indicates that cultural norms about eating and women's low social status often affect women's diets (Ransom, 2003). Some research has already been done on the correlation between gender and childhood malnutrition in different parts of the world. Most of these research shows that there is a relation between those two variables (Spears and Khera, 2013). Higher levels of gender inequality are associated with higher levels of undernutrition (Kshatriya, 2016). There is a strong correlation between a higher level of gender equality and lower level of child morbidity and mortality (FAO, 2013; Olofin, 2013).

Woman's status does influence child's nutritional status in three regions of the world: South Asia, Sub-Saharan Africa, and Latin America and the Caribbean (Smith, 2003). Evidence suggests that low social status of women in South Asia contributes to nutrition inequality (Shroff, 2011).

The prevalence of undernutrition and stunting among children under five years has declined globally but still remains high in South Asia (Black, 2013). About 46% of the children in South Asia are malnourished (The South Asia Food and Nutrition Security Problem, 2015). India has a high prevalence of undernutrition and a substantial level of gender disparity (Kshatriya, 2016). The prevalence of underweight in rural area is 50% versus 38% in urban area and higher among girls (48.9%) than boys (45.5%) (World Bank, 2014). Of the countries in South Asia, Bangladesh is the focus of this study due to its growing population and highest worldwide rate of chronic malnutrition; about 36% of the children were stunted and 33% were underweight (NIPORT, 2014). Female children are only slightly more likely to be underweight (33%) compared with male children (32%) (NIPORT, 2014). Bangladesh characterises many South Asian countries where women and girls experience inferiority in health and nutrition (Choudhury, 2000).

Various factors influence the rise in gender inequalities in nutrition. It is the consequence of food availability and dietary intake, breastfeeding, prevalence of infectious and parasitic diseases, access to health care, immunization gains, major childhood diseases, vitamin A supplementation, maternal care during pregnancy, water supply and sanitation, socioeconomic status, and health-seeking behaviour (Ndiku et al. 2011).

The present study aims to examine the association between socio-demographic and nutritional status of under five children with gender inequlity.

MATERIALS AND METHODS

This was a cross sectional and household level study. A multi-indicator survey design was prepared to explore a number of different and diverse issues related to health and nutrition among mothers and their preschool children. The proposed areas for this study were the rural areas in Rajshahi district of Bangladesh. Rajshahi is one of the highest poverty zones in Bangladesh (BBS, 2009). Around 2.3% ethnic minority representative, they are most deprived population (BBS, 2011).

In the present study, all children (aged 6-59 months) in the rural areas of Rajshahi district, Bangladesh were considered as the study population. The data was collected from the field survey conducted from October to December, 2016. All selected samples were interviewed by a group of expert researchers.

Sample Size Determination

The following mathematical formula was used to determine the sample size for this study:

$$n = \frac{N}{1 + Nd^2}$$

where, n = required sample size, N = household size (here 2,71,302), d = marginal error (we considered, $d = 0.05$), 95% confidence level (CI) had been considered (Yamane, 1967). The formula provided that the significant sample size was 399 for this study. Initially, we considered 540 under five children for this study.

Sample Selection Procedures

Multistage sampling technique was utilized to select samples covering all the population from all Upazilas of Rajshahi district. There are 9 Upazilas of Rajshahi district and in these Upazilas 232 Community Clinics (CCs) are running. In the first stage, 2 CCs had been selected from each Upazila by simple random sampling. A total of 18 (9 x 2) CCs were selected. In the second stage, 2 villages had been selected from each selected CC catchments areas by random sampling, total of 36 (18x2) villages were selected. In the third stage, 15 households had been selected from each selected village by random sampling which had at least one under five children. The children were identified by their identification number (holding number or listing). All information was got from respective Union Parishad (UP). If there was more than one mother in same household, one mother had been selected by lottery. If selected mother had more than one under five children, last born children was considered. A total of 540 under five children were considered as a sample in the present study.

Outcome Variables for These Children

Nutritional status was the outcome variable for the children. The following anthropometric measurements were used for calculating nutritional status of children (aged 6-59 months):

- Height for age (stunting) Z-score
- Weight for age (underweight) Z-score

Nutritional status was classified into three classes on the basis of z-scores, (i) under nutrition, (ii) healthy (normal), and (iii) over nutrition (WHO, 2006).

Independent Variables for This Study

The following socioeconomic, demographic, anthropometric, health and nutritional factors were considered as the independent variables with categories shown in the parenthesis:

Father's occupation (1: Farmers, 2: Labour, 3: business, 4: Service holder), Female headed household (1: Yes, 0: No), Father spent time at home (1: ≤ 3 hr, 2: ≥ 4 hr), Household food security (3 meal per day in last 12 month) (1: Yes, 0: No), Poverty status (1: Hardcore poor, 2 = Poor, 3 = Middle-rich), Children's Gender (1: Boys, 2: Girls), Children's age in months (1: 6-24 month; 2: 25-59 month), Mother's height in centimeter (1:≤ 145 cm, 2: > 145, Total household members (1: ≤3; 2: 4-5; 3: ≥6), Gestational at delivery [(≥37 week (full term), <37 week (pre-term)]. Mother received antenatal care (ANC) services (1: Yes, 0: No), Mother's antenatal care (ANC) visit during pregnancy (1: 1-3 visit, 2: 4 or more visit), Mother received tetanus toxoid (TT) injection during pregnancy (1: received TT injection, 0: No received), Mother took Iron-folic supplementation (IFS) during pregnancy (1:Yes, 0:No), Mother took vitamin A capsule (VAC) within six weeks of delivery (1: Yes, 0: No), Mother took extra food during pregnancy (1: Yes, 0: No), Mother took extra food during lactating (1: Yes, 0: No), Mother taken extra rest during pregnancy (1: Yes, 0: No).

Data Collection Method and Instruments

A partially structured and duly pre-tested questionnaire was used for collecting data from the respondents. First of all, a pilot survey was conducted in different study fields to observe whether there was any lacking or drawback in the questionnaire. After proper modification, questionnaire was finalized and made ready for data collection. The questionnaire was tested and validated by peers and other technical persons so as to ensure that the questions elicited the required answer. The questionnaires was pre-tested to check the length, content, question wording and language. The questionnaire was also pre-tested prior to data collection to ascertain content and face validity. Reliability refers to quality control measure of data collected. Before data collection, detailed study was based on the objectives of the study and on data collection techniques.

Data Processing and Management

The answered questionnaires were checked on a daily basis for accuracy and completeness in recoding of responses. Editing and coding was done before data entry. Data were entered and analyzed using SPSS (IBM version 20). The presence of abnormal point in data set, can affect the interpretation of results. The present author checked the outlier of the data set.

Statistical Analysis

Qualitative variables were explained with mean and standard deviation. Significant associations between two categorical variables were evaluated by applying relevant statistical tests (Chi square test) at appropriate probability level. Chi-square (χ^2)-test was used in this study to examine the association between children nutritional status and the selected socio-demographic variables. Significantly associated variables were considered as independent factors for further statistical model. Multiple logistic regression model was used to find the effect of socio-economic, demographic and health factors on malnutrition of the under five children. The results of the multiple logistic regression model were presented by adjusted odds ratio (AOR) with 95% confidence interval (CI) for the effects of the associated factors. Statistical significance was accepted at $p < 0.05$. Statistical analyses were carried out using SPSS software (IBM version 20).

RESULTS

Descriptive Statistics for Children (Aged 6-59 Months)

The descriptive statistics provide a useful description for data from any distribution, especially for variable with order and unordered categories. Mean and standard deviation of the children age, height and weight are presented in this section.

Table 1 exhibits the distribution of children (aged 6-59 months) by gender. It was noted that out of 540 children, the number of boys and girls were 273 (50.6%) and 267 (49.4%) respectively. More than 60% boys belonged to age group of 25-59 months and rest (38.10%) to 6-24 months, while 57.30% and 42.70% girls belonged to age groups of 25-59 months and 6-24 months respectively (Table 1).

Table 1. Distribution of children (aged 6-59 months) by gender

Age (in months)	**Gender**				**Total**	
	Boy		**Girl**			
	N	%	N	%	N	%
6-24	104	38.10	114	42.70	218	40.40
25-59	169	61.90	153	57.30	322	59.60
Total	273	50.55	267	49.45	540	100

N, the number of sample, %, percentage.

Table 2. Mean age, height and weight of children (aged 6-59 months) in the rural areas of Rajshahi district, Bangladesh

Variables	**Mean±SD**	**Mean±SD**	**MD**	**95% CI for MD**		**Total, 540**
	Boys, 273	**Girls, 267**		**Lower**	**Upper**	**Mean±SD**
Age (Month)	29.93 ± 14.69	29.50 ± 14.50	0.43	-2.04	2.90	29.72 ± 14.59
Height (cm)	83.49 ± 12.17	81.58 ± 12.24	1.91*	-0.16	3.97	82.55 ± 12.23
Weight (kg)	11.30 ± 3.08	10.68 ± 2.96	0.59*	0.08	1.10	10.98 ± 3.03

SD, Standard deviation; MD, Mean difference; CI, Confidence interval; *, 5% level of significance.

Table 2 shows the mean age, height and weight of children (aged 6-59 months) of the study area. It was observed that the mean age, height and weight of 540 children were 29.72 ± 14.58 months, 82.55 ± 12.23 cm and 10.98 ± 3.03 kg respectively. The mean age of boys and girls were 29.93 ± 14.69 month and 29.50 ± 14.50 month respectively, and the mean difference between two means was not statistically significant ($p > 0.05$). The mean height of boys (83.49 ± 12.17 cm) was higher than that of girls (81.58 ± 12.24 cm), and the difference between two values was statistically significant ($p < 0.05$). The mean weight of boys (11.30 ± 3.08 kg) was significantly higher than that of girls ($p < 0.05$).

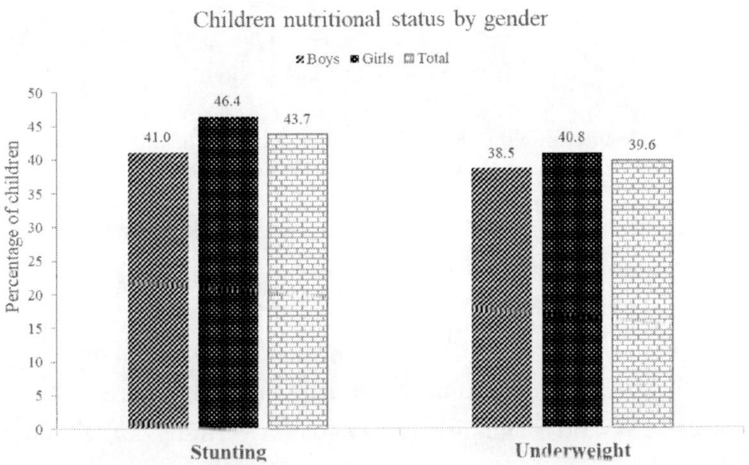

Figure 1. Nutritional status of children (aged 6-59 months) by gender.

Figure 1 displays the nutritional status of children (aged 6-59 months) by gender. The prevalence of stunting among children was 43.7%, and the prevalence among girls (46.4%) was higher than that among ~~of~~ boys (41.0%), z-proportion test demonstrated that the difference between these two proportions was not significant (p > 0.05). The prevalence of underweight among preschool children was 39.6%, and the prevalence among of girls (40.8%) was higher than that among of boys (38.5%), z-proportion test demonstrated that the difference between these two proportions was not significant (p > 0.05).

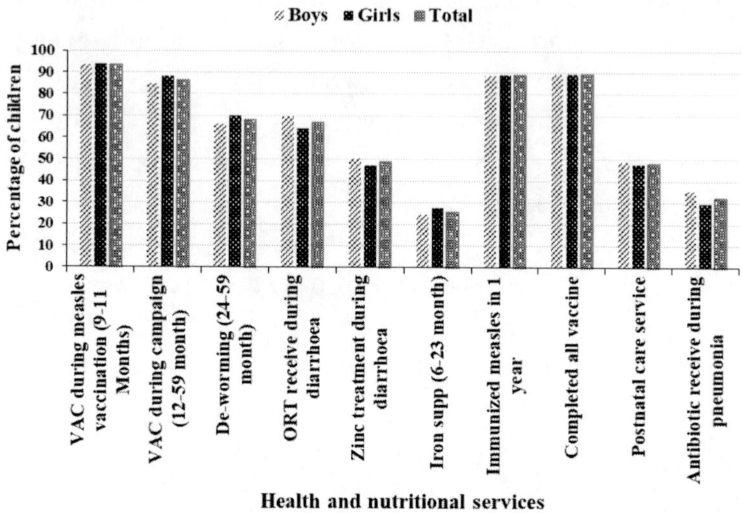

Figure 2. Prevalence of children (aged 6-59 months) received health and nutritional services by gender.

Figure 2 shows the prevalence of the health and nutritional services received by children (aged 6-59 months). About 94% children (boys, 93% and girls, 94%) received VAC during measles vaccination (infant's age 9-11 months) period, while 86% children (boys, 85% and girls, 88%) received the VAC during campaign (infant's age 12-59 months) period. More than 68% children (boys, 66% and girls, 70%) got de-worming tablet (in their age 24-59 months), while 67% (boys, 70% and girls, 64%) received oral rehydration therapy (ORT) during diarrhoea, and 49% (boys, 50% and girls, 47%) received zinc treatment during diarrhoea. More than 26% (boys, 24% and girls, 27%) received iron supplementation (in their age 6-23 months), while 89% (boys, 89% and girls, 89%) were immunized against measles in 1 year. It was noted that 89% (boys, 89% and girls, 90%) completed all vaccination. We observed that 48% (boys, 49% and girls, 48%) got postnatal care services and 32% (boys, 35% and girls, 30%) received antibiotic during pneumonia respectively (Figure 2).

Association between Nutritional Status of Children (Aged 6-59 Months) and Socio-Demographic Factors

Chi-square test ($\chi 2$) was used to determine the association between children nutritional status and socio-demographic factors (Table 3, 4 and 5).

For Stunting Children (Aged 6-59 Months)

In this study, it was found that stunting among boys (58.6%) was more than girls (56.2%) in a female headed household, and the association between female headed household and stunted status of boys was statistically significant ($p < 0.05$). Fathers who spent less time with their children (boys and girls) were more likely to get stunted children, the association between father spent time with their children and stunting status was statistically significant ($p < 0.01$). The study revealed that boys were more stunted in the food insecure households, and the association was statistically significant ($p < 0.01$) between two variables. It was investigated that girls (60.3%) who came from hardcore poor households were more likely to obtain stunting, and the association between girls stunted and poverty was statistically significant ($p < 0.05$). Short stature (height ≤145 cm) mother's daughters were more stunted than short stature mother's sons, and the association between girls stunted and short stature mothers was statistically significant ($p < 0.01$). This study found that girls (53.3%) who came from ≤3 members households were more stunted than boys (36.4%), and the association between girls stunted and total household members was statistically significant ($p < 0.01$). The full term (≥37 week) gestational age girls (48.9%) were more stunted than their counterparts (43.1%), and the association between girls stunted and gestation at delivery was statistically significant ($p < 0.05$).

Boys whose mothers didn't received antenatal care (ANC) services were more likely to get stunted than their counterparts, and the association between boys stunted and mother's receiving ANC services was statistically significant ($p < 0.01$). Mothers who didn't visit 4 or more ANC during their pregnancy period were more likely to get stunted children, and the association between two variables was statistically significant ($p < 0.01$). Mothers who didn't receive TT injection during their pregnancy were more likely to get stunted girls (51.1%) than boys (44.2%), and the association between stunting status of girls and mothers received TT injection during their pregnancy was statistically significant ($p < 0.05$). Mothers who didn't take iron-folic supplementation during pregnancy period were more likely to get stunted girls, and the association between stunted girls and mothers took iron-folic supplementation during pregnancy was statistically significant ($p < 0.01$). Mothers who didn't get extra food during lactating and extra rest during pregnancy had more chance to get stunted boys, and the association between two variables was statistically significant ($p < 0.05$).

For Underweight Children (Aged 6-59 Months)

This study found that fathers who's occupation were farmers had more chance to get underweightgirls (50.9%) than boys (43.3%), and the association between father's occupation of farming and stunted status of girls were statistically significant ($p < 0.05$). Fathers who spent less time with their children (boys and girls) were more likely to get underweight children, and the association between fathers spent time with their children and underweight status was statistically significant ($p < 0.05$).

The study revealed that girls were more underweight in the food insecure household, and the association was statistically significant ($p < 0.05$) between the two variables. It was investigated that girls (55.2%) who came from poor households had more chance to get underweight, and the association between girls underweight status and poverty was statistically significant ($p < 0.05$).

The full term (≥37 week) gestational age girls (43.7%) were more underweight than their counter parts (40.5%), and the association between girls underweight status and gestation at delivery was statistically significant ($p < 0.05$).

Table 3. Association between nutritional status of children and their parent's socioeconomic factors

Characteristics	Gender	Group (%)	Stunting (%)				Underweight (%)			
			Not stunted	Stunted	χ2	p-value	Not underweight	Underweight	χ2	p-value
Father's occupation	Boy	Farmer (41.4)	58.4	41.6	4.026	0.259	56.6	43.4	2.016	0.569
		Labour (35.9)	65.3	34.7			65.3	34.7		
		Business (16.1)	47.7	52.3			63.6	36.4		
		Service holder (6.6)	55.6	44.4			66.7	33.3		
	Girl	Farmer (41.9)	48.2	51.8	5.001	0.172	49.1	50.9	8.226	0.042
		Labour (35.2)	53.2	46.8			67.0	33.0		
		Business (14.6)	59.0	41.0			64.1	35.9		
		Service holder (8.2)	72.7	27.3			68.2	31.8		
Female headed household	Boy	Yes (10.6)	41.4	58.6	4.152	0.042	65.5	34.5	0.217	0.641
		No (89.4)	61.1	38.9			61.1	38.9		
	Girl	Yes (6.0)	43.8	56.2	0.658	0.417	62.5	37.5	0.078	0.780
		No (94.0)	54.2	45.8			59.0	41.0		
Father spent time at home	Boy	≤ 2 hour (42.5)	47.4	52.6	12.185	0.002	52.6	47.4	7.153	0.028
		3-5 hour (39.5)	64.8	35.2			66.7	33.3		
		≥ 6 hour (17.9)	73.5	26.5			71.4	28.6		
	Girl	≤hour (41.2)	43.6	56.4	20.658	0.001	46.4	53.6	14.886	0.001
		3-5 hour (36.0)	49.0	51.0			63.5	36.5		
		≥6 hour (22.8)	78.7	21.3			75.4	24.6		

Table 3. (Continued)

Characteristics	Gender	Group (%)	Stunting (%)				Underweight (%)			
			Not stunted	Stunted	χ2	p-value	Not underweight	Underweight	χ2	p-value
Household food security	Boy	No (11.0)	36.7	63.3	6.932	0.008	56.7	43.3	0.338	0.561
		Yes (89.0)	61.7	38.3			62.1	37.9		
	Girl	No (10.9)	44.8	55.2	0.997	0.318	37.9	62.1	6.078	0.014
		Yes (89.1)	54.6	45.4			61.8	38.2		
Poverty status	Boy	Poor (15.0)	58.5	41.5	4.829	0.089	63.4	36.6	1.951	0.377
		Middle (49.1)	53.0	47.0			57.5	42.5		
		Rich (35.9)	67.3	32.7			66.3	33.7		
	Girl	Poor (21.7)	39.7	60.3	5.872	0.053	44.8	55.2	7.429	0.024
		Middle (46.4)	56.5	43.5			66.1	33.9		
		Rich (31.8)	58.8	41.2			58.8	41.2		

Table 4. Association between nutritional status of children and demographic factors

Characteristics	Gender	Group	Stunting (%)				Underweight (%)			
			Not stunted	Stunted	χ2	p-value	Not underweight	Underweight	χ2	p-value
Children's age in months	Boy	6-24 (38.1)	51.9	48.1	3.452	0.063	52.9	47.1	5.316	0.021
		25-59 (61.9)	63.3	36.7			66.9	33.1		
	Girl	6-24 (42.7)	49.1	50.9	1.573	0.210	61.4	38.6	0.409	0.523
		25-59 (57.3)	56.9	43.1			57.5	42.5		
Mother's height in cm	Boy	≤ 145 (8.8)	41.7	58.3	3.258	0.071	54.2	45.8	0.604	0.437
		> 145 (91.2)	60.6	39.4			62.2	37.8		
	Girl	≤ 145 (13.9)	29.7	70.3	9.805	0.002	54.1	45.9	0.466	0.495
		> 145 (86.1)	57.4	42.6			60.0	40.0		
Total household members	Boy	≤3 (20.1)	63.6	36.4	2.734	0.255	58.2	41.8	1.061	0.588
		4-5 (55.7)	54.6	45.4			60.5	39.5		
		≥6 (24.2)	65.2	34.8			66.7	33.3		
	Girl	≤3 (22.5)	46.7	53.3	8.966	0.011	60.0	40.0	0.099	0.952
		4-5 (52.1)	48.9	51.1			58.3	41.7		
		≥6 (25.5)	69.1	30.9			60.3	39.7		
Gestational at delivery	Boy	≥37 week (full term) (85.0)	56.9	43.1	2.757	0.097	59.5	40.5	2.758	0.097
		<37 week (pre-term) (15.0)	70.7	29.3			73.2	26.8		
	Girl	≥37 week (full term) (85.8)	51.1	48.9	3.935	0.047	56.3	43.7	5.388	0.020
		<37 week (pre-term) (14.2)	68.4	31.6			76.3	23.7		

Table 5. Association between nutritional status of children and their mother's nutritional services

Characteristics	Gender	Group	Stunting (%)				Underweight (%)			
			Not stunted	Stunted	$\chi2$	p-value	Not underweight	Underweight	$\chi2$	p-value
Mother received ANC services	Boy	No (15.8)	76.7	23.3	6.661	0.010	55.8	44.2	0.707	0.401
		Yes (84.2)	55.7	44.3			62.6	37.4		
	Girl	No (15.7)	54.8	45.2	0.029	0.865	52.4	47.6	0.953	0.329
		Yes (84.3)	53.3	46.7			60.4	39.6		
Mother's ANC visit during pregnancy	Boy	1-3 visit (78.3)	49.4	50.6	12.928	0.001	58.9	41.1	4.894	0.027
		≥4 visit (21.7)	78.0	22.0			76.0	24.0		
	Girl	1-3 visit (77.8)	48.6	51.4	7.175	0.007	60.6	39.4	0.005	0.942
		≥4 visit (22.2)	70.0	30.0			60.0	40.0		
Mother received TT injection during pregnancy	Boy	No (63.0)	55.8	44.2	1.919	0.166	60.5	39.5	0.226	0.634
		TT (37.0)	64.4	35.6			63.4	36.6		
	Girl	No (65.9)	48.9	51.1	4.575	0.032	60.8	39.2	0.561	0.454
		TT (34.1)	62.6	37.4			56.0	44.0		
Mother took IFS during pregnancy	Boy	No (11.0)	53.3	46.7	0.443	0.506	50.0	50.0	1.896	0.169
		Yes (89.0)	59.7	40.3			63.0	37.0		
	Girl	No (7.9)	28.6	71.4	5.721	0.017	61.9	38.1	0.070	0.791
		Yes (92.1)	55.7	44.3			58.9	41.1		
Mother received VAC with six week of delivery	Boy	No (23.8)	52.3	47.7	1.567	0.211	49.2	50.8	5.460	0.019
		Yes (76.2)	61.1	38.9			65.4	34.6		
	Girl	No (20.6)	58.2	41.8	0.595	0.440	58.2	41.8	0.028	0.866
		Yes (79.4)	52.4	47.6			59.4	40.6		

Characteristics	Gender	Group	Stunting (%)				Underweight (%)			
			Not stunted	Stunted	$\chi2$	p-value	Not underweight	Underweight	$\chi2$	p-value
Mother took extra food during pregnancy	Boy	No (27.8)	51.3	48.7	2.553	0.110	51.3	48.7	4.650	0.031
		Yes (72.2)	61.9	38.1			65.5	34.5		
	Girl	No (26.6)	49.3	50.7	0.706	0.401	53.5	46.5	1.280	0.258
		Yes (73.4)	55.1	44.9			61.2	38.8		
Mother took extra food during lactating	Boy	No (26.7)	47.9	52.1	5.010	0.025	53.4	46.6	2.772	0.096
		Yes (73.3)	63.0	37.0			64.5	35.5		
	Girl	No (28.1)	56.0	44.0	0.250	0.617	57.3	42.7	0.147	0.702
		Yes (71.9)	52.6	47.4			59.9	40.1		
Mother taken extra rest during pregnancy	Boy	No (16.8)	43.5	56.5	5.491	0.019	52.2	47.8	2.050	0.152
		Yes (83.2)	62.1	37.9			63.4	36.6		
	Girl	No (20.2)	51.9	48.1	0.079	0.779	57.4	42.6	0.088	0.767
		Yes (79.8)	54.0	46.0			59.6	40.4		

Mothers who didn't visit 4 or more ANC during their pregnancy period were more likely to get underweight boys (41.1%) than their counterparts (39.4%), and the association between the two variables was statistically significant ($p < 0.01$). Mothers who didn't receive Vitamin A Capsule after six weeks of delivery were more likely to get underweight boys, and the association between underweight boys and mothers received Vitamin A Capsule after six weeks of delivery was statistically significant ($p < 0.05$). Mothers who didn't get extra food during pregnancy were more likely to get underweight boys, and the association between two variables was statistically significant ($p < 0.05$).

Effects of Socio-Demographic, Health and Nutritional Factors on Children Stunting and Underweight Status

All the significant associated factors were considered as independent variables for the multiple logistic regression model among stunted children (Table 6). The model demonstrated that fathers who spent ≥6 hours at home were less likely to have stunted boys than who spent less time (AOR = 0.360, 95% CI: 0.159-0.815; $p < 0.05$). Boys who came from female headed households were more likely to become stunted than their counterparts (AOR = 0.412, 95% CI: 0.173-0.983; $p < 0.05$). The mothers who didn't receive antenatal care services had more chance to have stunted boys than who received antenatal care services (AOR = 3.611, 95% CI: 1.537-8.487; $p < 0.01$). Girls who came from poor households were more likely to become stunted than their counterparts (AOR = 0.437, 95% CI: 0.195-0.978; $p < 0.05$). This study explored that short mothers (height ≤145cm) were more likely to have stunted girls than taller mothers (height > 145 cm) (AOR = 0.383, 95% CI: 0.163-0.900; $p < 0.05$). Girls who had ≥6 members household were less likely to become stunted than the girls living with less than 3 members household (AOR = 0.396, 95% CI: 0.175-0.896; $p < 0.05$). The mothers who didn't receive TT injection during pregnancy had more chance to have stunted girls than who received TT injection during pregnancy (AOR = 0.529, 95% CI: 0.284-0.985; $p < 0.05$).

Table 6. Effects of socio-demographic, health and nutrition factors on child stunting status

Gender	Independent variable	Coefficient (β)	S.E.	Wald	*p*-Value	Adjusted Odds Ratio (AOR)	95% CI of AOR
Boys	Father spent time at home						
	≤ 2 hour ®			7.186	0.028	1.00	
	3-5 hour	-0.624	0.313	3.964	0.046	0.536	0.290-0.990
	≥ 6 hour	-1.022	0.417	6.000	0.014	0.360	0.159-0.815
	Female headed household						
	Yes ®					1.00	
	No	-0.887	0.444	3.998	0.046	0.412	0.173-0.983
	Household food security (3 meal per day in last 12 month)						
	No ®					1.00	
	Yes	-0.306	0.479	0.408	0.523	0.736	0.288-1.883
	Poverty status						
	Poor®			3.107	0.212	1.00	
	Middle	0.595	0.424	1.972	0.160	1.812	0.790-4.157
	Rich	0.176	0.471	0.141	0.708	1.193	0.474-3.002
	Mother's height in cm						
	≤ 145 ®					1.00	
	> 145	-0.532	0.488	1.190	0.275	0.587	0.226-1.528
	Total household members						
	≤3 ®			1.325	0.515	1.00	
	4-5	0.329	0.364	0.812	0.367	1.389	0.680-2.837
	≥6	0.009	0.416	0.001	0.982	1.010	0.447-2.280

Table 6. (Continued)

Gender	Independent variable	Coefficient (β)	S.E.	Wald	*p*-Value	Adjusted Odds Ratio (AOR)	95% CI of AOR
	Gestational at delivery						
	≥37 week (full term) ®					1.00	
	<37 week (pre-term)	-0.459	0.401	1.311	0.252	0.632	0.288-1.387
	Mother received ANC services						
	No ®					1.00	
	Yes	1.284	0.436	8.678	0.003	3.611	1.537-8.487
	Mother received TT injection during pregnancy						
	No ®					1.00	
	Yes	-0.556	0.294	3.582	0.058	0.573	0.322-1.020
	Mother took Iron-folic supplementation during pregnancy						
	No ®					1.00	
	Yes	0.056	0.463	0.015	0.903	1.058	0.427-2.623
	Mother took extra food during lactating						
	No ®					1.00	
	Yes	-0.230	0.346	0.441	0.507	0.794	0.403-1.567
	Mother took extra rest during pregnancy						
	No®					1.00	
	Yes	-0.513	0.382	1.795	0.180	0.599	0.283-1.268
	Constant	0.761	0.976	0.607	0.436	2.139	

Gender	Independent variable	Coefficient (β)	S.E.	Wald	*p*-Value	Adjusted Odds Ratio (AOR)	95% CI of AOR
Girls	Father spent time at home						
	≤ 2 hour ®			12.925	0.002	1.00	
	3-5 hour	-0.259	0.334	0.600	0.439	0.772	0.401-1.485
	≥ 6 hour	-1.489	0.430	11.980	0.001	0.226	0.097-0.524
	Female headed household						
	Yes ®					1.00	
	No	-0.590	0.621	0.903	0.342	0.554	0.164-1.871
	Household food security (3 meal per day in last 12 month)						
	No ®					1.00	
	Yes	0.001	0.532	0.000	0.999	1.001	0.353-2.838
	Poverty status						
	Poor ®			4.086	0.130	1.00	
	Middle	-0.829	0.412	4.052	0.044	0.437	0.195-0.978
	Rich	-0.733	0.463	2.506	0.113	0.480	0.194-1.191
	Mother's height in cm						
	≤ 145 ®					1.00	
	> 145	-0.960	0.436	4.845	0.028	0.383	0.163-0.900
	Total household members						
	≤3 ®			5.180	0.075	1.00	

Table 6. (Continued)

Gender	Independent variable	Coefficient (β)	S.E.	Wald	*p*-Value	Adjusted Odds Ratio (AOR)	95% CI of AOR
	4-5	-0.339	0.363	0.873	0.350	0.712	0.350-1.451
	≥6	-0.925	0.416	4.943	0.026	0.396	0.175-0.896
	Gestational at delivery						
	≥37 week (full term) ®					1.00	
	<37 week (pre-term)	-0.412	0.442	0.869	0.351	0.662	0.278-1.576
	Mother received ANC services						
	No ®					1.00	
	Yes	0.248	0.395	0.393	0.531	1.281	0.590-2.779
	Mother received TT injection during pregnancy						
	No ®					1.00	
	Yes	-0.638	0.318	4.032	0.045	0.529	0.284-0.985
	Mother took Iron-folic supplementation during pregnancy						
	No ®					1.00	
	Yes	-1.205	0.564	4.564	0.033	0.300	0.099-0.905
	Mother took extra food during lactating						
	No ®					1.00	
	Yes	0.358	0.417	0.737	0.391	1.431	0.632-3.242
	Mother taken extra rest during pregnancy						
	No ®					1.00	
	Yes	0.719	0.474	2.302	0.129	2.052	0.811-5.192
	Constant	3.041	1.091	7.774	0.005	20.922	

Table 7. Effects of socio-demographic, health and nutrition factors on child underweight status

Gender	Independent variables	Coefficient (β)	S.E.	Wald	*p*-value	Adjusted Odds Ratio (AOR)	95% CI of AOR
Boys							
	Father spent time at home						
	≤ 2 hour ®			3.566	0.168	1.00	
	3-5 hour	-0.554	0.361	2.358	0.125	0.575	0.284-1.165
	≥ 6 hour	-0.803	0.478	2.818	0.093	0.448	0.175-1.144
	Father's occupation						
	Farmer ®			0.298	0.960	1.00	
	Labour	-0.079	0.350	0.051	0.821	0.924	0.465-1.834
	Business	-0.032	0.444	0.005	0.943	0.969	0.406-2.311
	Service holder	-0.329	0.627	0.275	0.600	0.720	0.211-2.458
	Household food security (3 meal per day in last 12 month)						
	No ®					1.00	
	Yes	0.576	0.512	1.268	0.260	1.779	0.653-4.849
	Poverty status						
	Poor ®			1.476	0.478	1.00	
	Middle	0.552	0.464	1.413	0.235	1.737	0.699-4.317
	Rich	0.395	0.535	0.544	0.461	1.484	0.520-4.236
	Children's age in months						
	6-24 ®					1.00	
	25-59	-0.637	0.301	5.193	0.023	0.503	0.279-0.908

Table 7. (Continued)

Gender	Independent variables	Coefficient (β)	S.E.	Wald	*p*-value	Adjusted Odds Ratio (AOR)	95% CI of AOR
	Gestational at delivery						
	≥37 week (full term) ®					1.00	
	<37 week (pre-term)	-0.616	0.457	1.819	0.177	0.540	0.221-1.322
	Mother's ANC visits during pregnancy						
	1-3 visit ®					1.00	
	4 or more visit	-0.706	0.394	3.211	0.073	0.494	0.228-1.068
	Mother received Vitamin A Capsule with six week of delivery						
	No ®					1.00	
	Yes	-0.613	0.346	3.127	0.077	0.542	0.275-1.069
	Mother took extra food during pregnancy						
	No ®					1.00	
	Yes	-0.443	0.350	1.598	0.206	0.642	0.323-1.276
	Constant	0.364	0.601	0.366	0.545	1.438	
Girls	Father spent time at home						
	≤ 2 hour ®			4.650	0.098	1.00	
	3-5 hour	-0.469	0.361	1.684	0.194	0.626	0.308-1.270
	≥ 6 hour	-0.960	0.448	4.588	0.032	0.383	0.159-0.922
	Father's occupation						
	Farmer ®			2.205	0.531	1.00	
	Labour	-0.390	0.355	1.205	0.272	0.677	0.338-1.358
	Business	-0.499	0.444	1.259	0.262	0.607	0.254-1.451
	Service holder	-0.623	0.615	1.026	0.311	0.537	0.161-1.790

Gender	Independent variables	Coefficient (β)	S.E.	Wald	*p*-value	Adjusted Odds Ratio (AOR)	95% CI of AOR
	Household food security (3 meal per day in last 12 month)						
	No ®					1.00	
	Yes	-0.499	0.543	0.844	0.358	0.607	0.210-1.760
	Poverty status						
	Poor ®			3.051	0.218	1.00	
	Middle	-0.526	0.419	1.579	0.209	0.591	0.260-1.343
	Rich	0.036	0.480	0.006	0.940	1.037	0.404-2.659
	Children's age in months						
	6-24 ®					1.00	
	25-59	-0.051	0.290	0.031	0.860	0.950	0.538-1.678
	Gestational at delivery						
	≥37 week (full term) ®					1.00	
	<37 week (pre-term)	-0.487	0.491	0.985	0.321	0.614	0.235-1.608
	Mother's ANC visits during pregnancy						
	1-3 visit ®					1.00	
	4 or more visit	-0.014	0.359	0.002	0.969	0.986	0.488-1.992
	Mother received Vitamin A Capsule with six week of delivery						
	No ®					1.00	
	Yes	0.027	0.390	0.005	0.946	1.027	0.478-2.205
	Mother took extra food during pregnancy						
	No ®					1.00	
	Yes	-0.008	0.364	0.001	0.982	0.992	0.486-2.024
	Constant	0.962	0.590	2.661	0.103	2.618	

The mothers who didn't take iron-folic supplementation during pregnancy had more chance to have stunted girls than who took iron-folic supplementation during pregnancy (AOR = 0.300, 95% CI: 0.099-0.905; $p < 0.05$).

Again, all the associated factors were considered as independent variables for the multiple logistic regression model among underweight children (Table 7). The model demonstrated that boys aged 6-24 months had more chance to have underweight than their counterparts (AOR = 0.503, 95% CI: 0.279-0.908; $p < 0.05$). Fathers who spent ≥ 6 hours at home were less likely to have underweight girls than who spent at home less than ≤ 2 hours (AOR = 0.383, 95% CI: 0.159-0.922; $p < 0.05$).

DISCUSSION

In this study, we investigated association of nutritional status and socio-demographic factors among the children aged 6-59 months in Rajshahi district of Bangladesh in relation to gender inequality. In BDHS 2014, 31.1% children were found stunted and 32.1% underweight in Rajshahi division. Our study revealed that 43.7% children were stunted and 39.6% underweight in this rural area, compared to national rate of 36% stunted and 33% underweight. According to BDHS 2014, Stunting is slightly higher among boys (36.7%) than among girls (35.4%). And underweight is slightly higher among girls (33.1) than among boys (32.2%). In this survey, data showed that rates of both stunted and underweight were higher among the girls (46.4% and 40.8%) than boys (41.0% and 38.5%) respectively. Data clearly showed that gender inequality exists regarding nutritional status among children of under five years in Bangladesh.

A study (Haidar, 2009) found that the prevalence of stunted and underweight among under-five children was significantly higher in female-headed households than in the male-headed households. Our study showed similar results but it was found statistically significant only among boys.

The majority (42.5%) of the fathers spent ≤2 hours at home each day with their children. We found it has impact stunted and underweight status of children (boys and girls), the association of the two variables is statistically significant among both girls ($p < 0.001$) and boys ($p < 0.02$). Girls suffer from stunting and underweight more compared to boys. Similar results were found by Jesmin in Bangladesh (2011).

Fathers' occupation has impact on girls underweight. data showed that girls are more underweight (50.9%) than boys (43.45). Poverty and household food security were two important factors related to the prevalence of stunting and underweight among boys (38.3% and (41.5%) and girls (45.4% and 60.3%) respectively. we found alike results in Ethiopia (Mulu, 2017) and India (Kshatriya, 2016).

Extra food taken during pregnancy of mother has impact on children stunted status showing that girl's mothers took less extra food during their pregnancy. Similar findings were also found in India (Mishra, 2004) and Ethiopia (Nigatu, 2018).

This study explored that short stature mothers (height ≤145cm) were more likely to have stunted girls with comparison to boys. Similar result was found in low-to middle-income countries (Özaltin, 2010). Girls were more stunted in the small family size households, which implies that cares towards girls get less priorities.

Mother having ANC service and frequent visit has impact on children stunting and underweight. Hemel in Nigeria (2015), Talukder in Bangladesh (2017) and Nigatu in Ethiopia (2018) found similar results. The likelihoods of underweight and stunting in this study were high among mothers who had less or no antenatal care services. This might be due to the fact that access to health care services, like ANC, is important sources of information for pregnant women to get nutritional and health messages. Girls of the mothers who didn't receive TT injection during her pregnancy are more stunted in comparison to boys.

Limitation of the Study

The present study has some limitations. First of all, the data were collected from the rural area of north-western district in Bangladesh. Secondly, this study didn't take some important variables into consideration that might affect the nutritional status of children such as dietary aspects and biochemical tests at individual level. While conducting the interviews, we had to depend on the information provided by mothers. Information could, thus, have been subject to recall bias. However, we were careful in recording the information they provided and in the interpretation of the results of the study.

Conclusion

A total number of 540 under five children were considered from the rural area of Rajshahi district to investigate the association between socio-demographic and children nutritional status with gender differentiates. Descriptive statistics, Chi-sqaure test and binary logistic regression model were used to analyse the data. Our selected statistical models provided that boys had better nutritional status compared with girls. Though gender inequality is reduceing in Bangladesh but it exists significantly in rural areas. Socio-demographic and nutritional service factors had positive impact on nutritional status but study revealed that still there was gender imbalance. Gender inequalities in nutrition were considered important factors that undermine efforts to achieve sustainable development. It was observed that the socio-cultural nature of the inferior position of women in this rural society was important predictor. It was suggested that broad-based interventions would be needed to improvegirls' health and nutritional status.

References

Addo, O. Y., Stein, A. D., Fall, C. H., Gigante, D. P., Guntupalli, A. M., Horta, B. L., & Richter, L. M. (2013). Maternal height and child growth patterns. *The Journal of pediatrics*, 163(2), 549-554.

Abdi, N., Sadeghi, R., Zamani-alavijeh, F., Taghdisi, M. H., &Shojaeezadeh, D. (2016). Explaining nutritional habits and behaviors of low socioeconomic status women in Sanandaj: a qualitative content analysis. *Electronic physician*, 8(1), 1733.

Assan, N. (2013). Women empowerment as a tool against food insecurity in Sub Saharan Africa. *A Review. Sci. J. Rev*, 2(11), 329-339.

Assembly, U. G. (2015). Transforming our world: the 2030 Agenda for Sustainable Development. *New York: United Nations*, (1).

BBS, WFP and World Bank. (2009). Poverty Maps of Bangladesh 2010. *Bangladesh Bureau of Statistics* and World Food Programme and World Bank, Dhaka. Available, at: https://www.wfp.org/sites/default/files/Poverty%20Map%202010_Key%20Findings_BBS%20WB%20WFP.pdf.

BBS. (2011). Population and Housing Census 2011. *Bangladesh Bureau of Statistics*. Statistics and Informatics Division, Ministry of Planning. Government of the People's Republic of Bangladesh.

Balgir, R. S. (2009). Impact of gender bias on health and nutrition of the tribal women in relation to dynamics of development in India. *Internet Journal of Biological Anthropology*, 3(1): 1-6.

Betebo, B., Ejajo, T., Alemseged, F., & Massa, D. (2017). Household food insecurity and its association with nutritional status of children 6–59 months of age in east Badawacho District, south Ethiopia. *Journal of environmental and public health*, 2017.

Bender, D. A. (2009). *A dictionary of food and nutrition*. OUP Oxford.

Black, R. E., Victora, C. G., Walker, S. P., Bhutta, Z. A., Christian, P., De Onis, M., & Uauy, R. (2013). Maternal and child undernutrition and overweight in low-income and middle-income countries. *The lancet*, 382(9890), 427-451.

Bose, S. (2011). The effect of women's status and community on the gender differential in children's nutrition in India. *Journal of biosocial science*, 43(5), 513-533.

Bredenkamp, C., Buisman, L. R., & Van de Poel, E. (2014). Persistent inequalities in child undernutrition: evidence from 80 countries, from 1990 to today. *International Journal of Epidemiology*, 43(4), 1328-1335.

Choudhury, K. K., Hanifi, M. A., Rasheed, S., & Bhuiya, A. (2000). Gender inequality and severe malnutrition among children in a remote rural area of Bangladesh. *Journal of Health, Population and Nutrition*, 123-130.

Coffey, D., Khera, R., & Spears, D. (2013). Women's status and children's height in India: Evidence from joint rural households. Unpublished, Office of Population Research, Wallace Hall, Princeton University, Princeton, NJ, 8540.

Commission on the Social Determinants of Health (CSDH). (2008). Closing the gap in a generation: Health equity through action on the social determinants of health, *final report of the commission on social determinants of health*, WHO.

Dey, I., & Chaudhuri, R. N. (2008). Gender inequality in nutritional status among underfive children in a village in Hooghly district, West Bengal. *Indian J Public Health*, 52(4), 218-20.

Dancer, D., Rammohan, A., & Smith, M. D. (2008). Infant mortality and child nutrition in Bangladesh. *Health economics*, 17(9), 1015-1035.

FAO, A. (2013). Gender Equality and Food Security–Women's empowerment as a Tool against Hunger. Mandaluyong City, Philippines: *ADB*. ISBN 978-92-9254-172-9.

FAO (2015). *Women play a decisive role in household food security, dietary diversity and children's health.*

Haidar, J., & Kogi-Makau, W. (2009). Gender differences in the household-headship and nutritional status of pre-school children. *East African medical journal*, 86(2).

Hannan, A. *The Association between Women's Empowerment and Child Nutrition in Bangladesh*.

Hamel, C., Enne, J., Omer, K., Ayara, N., Yarima, Y., Cockcroft, A., & Andersson, N. (2015). Childhood malnutrition is associated with maternal care during pregnancy and childbirth: a cross-sectional study in Bauchi and Cross River States, Nigeria. *Journal of Public Health Research*, 4:408. doi:10.4081/jphr.2015.408.

Jawaregowda, S. K., & Angadi, M. M. (2015). Gender differences in nutritional status among under five children in rural areas of Bijapur district, Karnataka, India. *International Journal of Community Medicine and Public Health*, 2(4), 506-509.

Jesmin, A., Yamamoto, S. S., Malik, A. A., &Haque, M. A. (2011). Prevalence and determinants of chronic malnutrition among preschool children: a cross-sectional study in Dhaka City, Bangladesh. *Journal of Health, Population, and Nutrition*, 29(5):494-499.

Kshatriya, G. K., &Acharya, S. K. (2016). Gender Disparities in the Prevalence of Undernutrition and the Higher Risk among the Young Women of Indian Tribes. *PloS one*, 11(7), e0158308. doi:10.1371/journal.pone.0158308.

Marphatia, A. A., Cole, T. J., Grijalva-Eternod, C., & Wells, J. C. (2016). Associations of gender inequality with child malnutrition and mortality across 96 countries. *Global health, epidemiology and genomics*, 1.

Mishra, V., Roy, T. K., & Retherford, R. D. (2004). Sex differentials in childhood feeding, health care, and nutritional status in India. *Population and development review*, 30(2), 269-295.

Moestue, H. (2009). Can anthropometry measure gender discrimination? An analysis using WHO standards to assess the growth of Bangladeshi children. *Public health nutrition*, 12(8), 1085-1091.

Mucha, N. (2012). Enabling and equipping women to improve nutrition. *Briefing Paper*, (16), Bread for the World Institute, Washington D.C.

Mulu, E., & Mengistie, B. (2017). Household food insecurity and its association with nutritional status of under five children in Sekela District, Western Ethiopia: a comparative cross-sectional study. *BMC Nutrition*, 3(1), 35.

Ndiku, M., Jaceldo Siegl, K., Singh, P., &Sabate, J. (2011). Gender inequality in food intake and nutritional status of children under 5 years old in rural Eastern Kenya. *European journal of clinical nutrition*, 65(1), 26.

Nigatu, G., Woreta, S. A., Akalu, T. Y., &Yenit, M. K. (2018). Prevalence and associated factors of underweight among children 6–59 months of age in Takusa district, Northwest Ethiopia. *International journal for equity in health*, 17(1), 106.

National Institute of Population Research and Training (NIPORT). (2014). *Bangladesh Demographic and Health Survey 2014*. Dhaka, Bangladesh and Rockville, Maryland, USA: NIPORT, Mitra and Associates, and ICF International.

Nigatu, G., Woreta, S. A., Akalu, T. Y., & Yenit, M. K. (2018). Prevalence and associated factors of underweight among children 6–59 months of age in Takusa district, Northwest Ethiopia. *International journal for equity in health*, 17(1), 106.

Olofin, I., McDonald, C. M., Ezzati, M., Flaxman, S., Black, R. E., Fawzi, W. W., & Nutrition Impact Model Study (anthropometry cohort pooling. (2013). Associations of suboptimal growth with all-cause and cause-specific mortality in children under five years: a pooled analysis of ten prospective studies. *PloS one*, 8(5), e64636.

Özaltin, E., Hill, K., & Subramanian, S. V. (2010). Association of maternal stature with offspring mortality, underweight, and stunting in low-to middle-income countries. *Jama*, 303(15), 1507-1516.

Shroff, M. R., Griffiths, P. L., Suchindran, C., Nagalla, B., Vazir, S., & Bentley, M. E. (2011). Does maternal autonomy influence feeding practices and infant growth in rural India? *Social science & medicine*, 73(3), 447-455.

Smith, L. C. (Ed.). (2003). The importance of women's status for child nutrition in developing countries (Vol. 131). *Intl Food Policy Res Inst*. Washington, DC.

Talukder, A. (2017). Factors associated with malnutrition among under-five children: illustration using Bangladesh demographic and health survey, 2014 data. *Children*, 4(10), 88.

Tigga, P. L., Debnath, S., Das, M., Mondal, N., Sen, J. (2018). Prevalence of undernutrition and overweight or obesity among the Bengali Muslim population of West Bengal, India. *Anthropol Open J*. 2018; 3(1): 1-10. doi: 10.17140/ANTPOJ-3-115.

The South Asia Food and Nutrition Security Problem. (2015). Retrieved September 15, 2015, from World Bank: http://web.worldbank.org/WBSITE/EXTERNAL/COUNTRIES/SOUTHASIAEXT/0,,contentMDK:22826499~pagePK:146736~piP:146830~theSitePK:223547,00.html.

UNICEF. (2011). Gender influences on child survival, health and nutrition: a narrative review. *New York*.

UNICEF, WHO, World Bank Group (2015). Levels and trends in child malnutrition, key findings of the 2015 edition. Retrieved from http://www.who.int/nutrition/publications/jointchildmalnutrition_2015_estimates/en/.

Vlassoff, C. (2007). Gender differences in determinants and consequences of health and illness. *Journal of health, population, and nutrition*, 25(1), 47.

World Health Organization. (2006). WHO child growth standards: length/height-for-age, weight-for-age, weight-for-length, weight-for-height and body mass index-for-age. Methods and Development. *WHO* (nonserial publication). Geneva: WHO, 2007. Available at: http://www.who.int/childgrowth/standards/technical_report/en/.

World Health Organization. (2015). Gender, Fact sheet N° 403, Updated August 2015. Retrieved from http://who.int/mediacentre/factsheets/fs403/en/.

World Health Organization. (2017). Guideline: assessing and managing children at primary health-care facilities to prevent overweight and obesity in the context of the double burden of malnutrition. Updates for the Integrated Management of Childhood Illness (IMCI). Geneva: *World Health Organization*; 2017. Licence: CC BY-NC-SA 3.0 IGO.

World Health Organization. (2018). http://www.who.int/en/news-room/fact-sheets/detail/malnutrition.

Wood, J. (2005). *Gendered Lives*, 6th. Belmont, CA: Wadsworth/Thomson Learning.

World Bank. (2006). *Repositioning nutrition as central to development a strategy for large-scale action.* Directions in Development (EUA). Washington DC: USA. Available online at http://siteresources.worldbank.org/NUTRITION/Resources/281846-1131636806329/NutritionStrategy.pdf. Accessed 15 September 2009.

World Bank. (2014). Undernourished. Chapter 1. What Are The Dimensions Of The Undernutrition Problem In India? [Internet].2014 [cited 2014 August 20]. Available from http://siteresources.worldbank.org/SOUTHASIAEXT/Resources/223546 1147272668285/undernourished_chapter_1.pdf.

Yamane, Taro. 1967. *Statistics, An Introductory Analysis*, 2nd Ed., New York: Harper and Row.

In: Contemporary Issues in Childhood … ISBN: 978-1-53617-348-2
Editors: J. Ratan Ghosh and K. Bose

Chapter 3

POLIO IMMUNIZATION AND MALNUTRITION

***Jaydip Sen*[1,*]*, PhD and Shreyasi Roy*[1,†]**

[1]Department of Anthropology, University of North Bengal, West Bengal, India

ABSTRACT

Vaccination (or rather immunization) is considered a breakthrough in preventive medicine. Vaccination at age-appropriate intervals increases protection against morbidity and mortality since childhood through various recommended vaccination schedules. The question still prevails whether all those vaccinated children are really immunized. The present paper deals with this issue. The paper presents an overview on various studies that clearly depicted that malnourished children are suffering the ineffective-ness of polio vaccine.

---

[*]Correponding Author's Email: jaydipsen@rediffmail.com.
[†] Corresponding Author's Email: shreyasiroy93@gmail.com.

INTRODUCTION

Vaccinations are a boost to our immune system. Its origin dates back to 1796 when Edward Jenner residing in Berkeley (Gloucestershire), England developed the world's first vaccine (Baxby, 1981). His groundbreaking discovery has resulted today in defending the human body against various diseases like chickenpox, diphtheria, hepatitis A, hepatitis B, influenza, measles, meningococcal, mumps, pneumococcal, polio, rotavirus, rubella, shingles, tetanus, etc. Despite having minor side-effects like fatigue, headache, nausea, dizziness, low-grade fever, fussiness and soreness where the vaccine shot is administered, vaccinations are considered to be the safest method of safeguarding an individual from various devastating diseases. Various organizations and institutes like Centers for Disease Control and Prevention (CDC), World Health Organization (WHO), American Academy of Pediatrics (AAP), Indian Academy of Pediatrics (IAP) and National Rural Health Mission (NRHM) by Government of India aim to provide immunity to an individual from early life through recommended vaccination schedule. One such fatal disease named Poliomyelitis (commonly called polio) is thought to be prevented (rather than cured because it is non-curable) through routinely vaccination starting after birth.

The words "polio" (grey) and "myelon" (marrow, indicating the spinal cord) are derived from Greek (Chamberlin and Narins, 2005). Hence, it could be inferred that 'poliomyelitis' (often called polio) is one of the dreadful diseases which invades the nervous system of the individual and can cause permanent and/or irreversible paralysis in <1% of infected individuals (Baicus, 2012). As a result, this acute viral disease is also known as 'infantile paralysis.' It is a highly contagious disease which usually spreads through faeco-oral route, droplet infection or less often by a common channel that is polluted food or water (Atkinson et al., 2009).

To combat this fatal disease, two types of vaccines have been employed so far. In early 1950s, the first polio vaccine was developed called inactivated poliovirus vaccine (IPV) or Salk vaccine (as it was developed by Jonas Salk). This vaccine is based on three virulent reference strains - Mahoney (type 1 poliovirus), MEF-1 (type 2 poliovirus), and Saukett (type

3 poliovirus) and is given by intramuscular or intra-dermal injection. The second one called oral polio vaccine (OPV) which is a live attenuated vaccine developed by Albert Sabin.

Could We Really Prepare a Polio-Free World?

Despite several attempts, it is unfortunate that we could not make our world polio-free till date. The goal of global eradication of poliomyelitis was adopted in 1988 and since then Global Polio Eradication Initiative (GPEI) has reduced the occurrence of polio worldwide by almost 99% except few failures. Three countries, i.e., Afghanistan, Pakistan and Nigeria still have frequent outbreaks of wild polio virus and are still considered epidemic to this fatal disease (Ado et al., 2014; Kew et al., 2014; Hagan et al., 2015; Moeti 2016; Shah et al., 2016; Mahmood, 2018; Martinez et al., 2018). India was removed from the list of polio-endemic countries by 'Polio-free certification of the World Health Organization South-East Asia Region' in the year 2014. Thus, the strong urge and planned attempts of GPEI, WHO, CDC, Rotary foundation and other health institutes were able to make a huge shift from an estimated 350,000 polio cases in 125 countries to approximately 512 cases in just 3 countries during the period of 3 decades (1988-2018).

The GPEI has preferred to rely on oral poliovirus vaccine (OPV) rather than inactivated vaccine, primarily because of its superior ability to induce gut mucosal immunity (Ghendon and Sanakoyeva, 1961; WHO, 2008). Additionally, OPV is cheaper than IPV and can be easily orally administered (WHO, 2013). It has a herd effect, inducing long-lasting protective systemic, humoral and cellular immunity as well as local mucosal resistance to polio virus infection (Baicus, 2012).In polio-endemic countries and in areas at high risk for importation and subsequent spread, WHO (2017) recommends an OPV dose at birth (called 'zero' dose), followed by the primary series of three OPV doses with at least one IPV dose.

Being a comparatively better and more reliable solution, OPV had been used in routine immunization and in supplementary immunization activities throughout the polio eradication initiative. However, the immunogenicity of OPV was found to be lower in some developing countries with seroconversion rates less than 40% (Hamer, 2010; Jafari et al., 2014) as compared to developed and industrialized ones with seroconversion rates greater than 80% (Cáceres and Sutter, 2001). On being questioned, several hypotheses like malnutrition, diarrheal disease and environmental enteropathy came up as the reason for OPV failure (John, 1975; Myaux et al., 1996; Zaman et al., 2009; Korpe and Petri, 2012).

Could Malnutrition Be a Cause of OPV Failure?

Though the term 'malnutrition' comprises both under-nutrition and over-nutrition, it is said to be equivalent to only under-nutrition unless anything is specified. Malnutrition is the common issue prevalent in developing and underdeveloped countries (Müller and Krawinkel, 2005), and also in developed countries to some extent. It contributes to more than half of deaths among children of less than 5 years of age (Caulfield et al., 2004). There exists several contributing factors in childhood malnutrition, some of which are low birth weight, inadequate breast feeding and exclusive breastfeeding, inappropriate complementary feeding, maternal education, lack of proper knowledge of nutrition, micronutrient intake, parity, birth spacing, household socioeconomic status, food insecurity, poor sanitation, vaccination, and infectious diseases (Jesmin et al., 2011; Lozano et al., 2012; Engell and Lim, 2013; Guerrant et al., 2013; Wolf et al., 2014).

Earlier, studies of Greenwood et al. (1986) and Chopra et al. (1989) claimed that mild and moderately malnourished children were most often found to seroconvert normally when vaccinated against polio. However, according to WHO (2013), malnutrition is the root cause of failure of all vaccinations. According to few data from WHO, it was highlighted that malnutrition hinders the battle against polio because OPV produces four times less immunity in malnourished children as compared to well-nourished (Yousuf et al., 2015). In a study by Haque et al. (2014), an association of diminished immunogenicity of OPV type 3 virus with undernutrition as well as with shorter duration of exclusive breastfeeding has been found. On the other hand, no association was found between IPV immunogenicity and these variables which further conclude that OPV is less effective in developing as well as underdeveloped countries where these variables are almost common.

Low birth weight (less than 2500 gm measured at the first hour after birth) and preterm (gestation period less than 37 weeks) are some of the root causes of childhood malnutrition. Although it has been recommended by the American Academy of Pediatrics Committee on Infectious Diseases (1988) that premature children must receive immunizations at the same chronological age as full-term children, primary care physicians and parents remain hesitant to immunize preterm children who have complex medical histories. Most of them mistakenly believe that other factors such as birth weight, current weight, or degree of prematurity should influence the timing of immunizations for preterm children (Langkamp and Langhough, 1992; 1993). Hence, even though preterm children and low birth weight babies can mount adequate immune responses when immunized at the recommended chronological age, they often receive immunizations on a delayed schedule (Vohr and Oh, 1986). Furthermore, majority of maternal IgG antibodies gets transferred to an infant *in utero* usually during the final trimester which is often missed by preterm babies and this makes them prone to various sorts of infection. Hence, timely vaccination including booster doses is a must to these babies as they are devoid of passive immunity before vaccination (Okoko et al., 2001) and may respond sub-optimally to primary vaccination (Baxter, 2010). It has also been observed that extremely premature infants have diminished responsiveness to serotype 3 polio vaccine (D'Angio et al., 1995).

Dietary factors play a role in the antibody response of infants to immunization (Pickering et al., 1998). Feeding human milk was observed to enhance antibody response to OPV (Pickering et al., 1998). Infants who were breastfed had significantly higher neutralizing antibody titers to polio virus than either formula-fed group at 6 months of age (Pickering et al., 1998). Similarly, another study by Hahn-Zoric et al. (1990) concluded that breastfed infants showed better serum and secretory responses to peroral and parenteral vaccines than the formula-fed.

Probable Causes

There are several hypotheses stating the cause of the association of malnutrition (more specifically, under-nutrition) and OPV failure. Infections resulting from malnutrition enhance the severity of malnutrition further, generating a positive vicious cycle which in turn affects most aspects of immune system of the body (Bendich and Deckelbaum, 2009). This may affect cell-mediated immunity more compared to humoral immunity (Gershwin et al., 2004). Moreover, severe under-nutrition causes atrophy of lymphoid organs, decrease in the bone marrow reserves of leukocyte, decrease in proliferative response of T lymphocytes to antigens, and decrease in natural killer cell activity (Gershwin et al., 2004). Protein-energy malnutrition is found to be associated with reduction of regulatory immune responses in the mucosal microenvironment which potentially impairs the mechanisms of oral tolerance (Campbell et al., 2003).

How Can We Prevent This?

A world without polio is an unfulfilled dream to many researchers. Malnutrition is a major determinant of the humoral response to oral polio vaccines and must be given due consideration to prevent vaccination failure (Caidi et al., 2004). In order to accelerate poliovirus eradication, it is important to focus on the lowest socioeconomic strata of society where malnutrition is most prevalent (Hussain et al., 2017).

Supplementation during polio campaigns or from health centers can surely reduce the deficiency of various nutrients and can aid to improve the efficacy of polio vaccine, especially OPV. In a study by Cobra et al. (1997), oral iodized oil supplementation has been shown to improve infant survival in a clinical trial in Indonesia in which infants received oral iodized oil or placebo immediately after their first dose of OPV. Furthermore, it was claimed by Taffs et al. (1999) that supplementation with oral iodized oil may be safely combined with delivery of the first dose of OPV in the Expanded Programme on Immunization (EPI) schedule as this does not reduce neutralizing antibody responses to OPV. However, no effect of zinc supplementation on OPV immunogenicity was found (Habib et al., 2015). The same was seen in the case of vitamin A supplementation among infants during the EPI centers where this supplementation imposed no effect on infants' antibody responses to oral polio vaccine as well as on their seroconversion rates (Newton et al., 2005; Rahman et al., 1997). However, the administration of vitamin A supplements during the polio immunization days is considered as one of the effective methods to eliminate the risk of subclinical vitamin A deficiency (Goodman et al., 2000). Besides this, adequate levels of vitamin A are required for optimal antibody responses and other immune functions (Ross, 1992).

IPV given with OPV induced superior immune responses than OPV alone in well-nourished and malnourished infants in Pakistan (Saleem et al., 2015). This was earlier proved by WHO collaborative study group (1997) where a clinical trial was conducted among the children of countries like Gambia, Oman, and Thailand. The study found that the combined schedule of IPV and OPV provided the highest levels of serum antibody response, with mucosal immunity equivalent to that produced by OPV alone.

In low-income countries, seroconversion rates were found to be suboptimal following administration of three-dose tOPV regimens (Patriarca et al., 1991; Khare et al., 1993; Grassly et al., 2010). These rates were found to approach nearly 100 % in many industrialized countries. The findings of Sutter et al. (2010) and few other studies exhibited the superiority of bivalent oral poliovirus vaccine (bOPV) compared with trivalent oral poliovirus vaccine (tOPV). Hence, in April 2016, the WHO implemented a worldwide switch from tOPV to a bOPV removing live poliovirus serotype 2 from global use (Sutter et al., 2014). In addition, the study of Grassly et al. (2006) attempted to show that switching to monovalent vaccine may finally interrupt polio virus transmission. Sutter et al. (2010) displayed the non-inferiority of bOPV compared with mOPV1 and mOPV3 which is consistent with the study of O'Reilly et al. (2012) that interpreted that the effectiveness of bOPV is comparable with that of mOPV.

Conclusion

Polio is a dreadful disease which needs to be eradicated from all parts of the world. Owing to several factors, this disease still prevails in many of the countries till date. One such factor is "childhood malnutrition" which hinders the battle against this disease. More studies need to be conducted on how to combat childhood malnutrition and associated causes. Studies need to be done on to improve the effectiveness of polio vaccine worldwide.

References

Ado JM, Etsano A, Shuaib F, Damisa E, Mkanda P, Gasasira A, Banda R, Korir C, Johnson T, Dieng B, Corkum M, Enemaku O, Mataruse N, Ohuabunwo C, Baig S, Galway M, Seaman V, Wiesen E, Vertefeuille J, Ogbuanu IU, Armstrong G, Mahoney FJ. 2014. Progress toward poliomyelitis eradication in Nigeria. *J. Infect. Dis.* 210 Suppl. 1:S40-S49.

American Academy of Pediatrics Committee on Infectious Diseases. 1988. The 1988 Red Book, 21st ed. Elk Grove Village, *Ill American Academy of Pediatrics*. p. 323-324.

Atkinson W, Hamborsky J, McIntyre L, Wolfe S, 2009. Poliomyelitis: Epidemiology and Prevention of Vaccine-Preventable Diseases, 11th ed. Washington DC, *Public Health Foundation*. p. 231-44.

Baicus A. 2012. History of polio vaccination. *World J. Virol.* 1:108-114.

Baxby D, 1981. Jenner's Smallpox Vaccine: The Riddle of Vaccinia Virus and Its Origin. London, *Heinemann Educational Books*.

Baxter D. 2010.Vaccine responsiveness in premature infants. *Hum. Vaccin.* 6(6):506-511.

Bendich A, Deckelbaum RJ, 2009. *Preventive nutrition: the comprehensive guide for health professionals,* 4th ed. New York, Humana Pr Inc.

Cáceres VM, Sutter RW. 2001. Sabin monovalent oral polio vaccines: review of past experiences and their potential use after polio eradication. *Clin. Infect. Dis*. 33(4):531-541.

Caidi H, Bennis IF, Mouan N, El Aouad R. 2004.Evaluation of the response to vaccination against poliomyelitis and measles in malnourished children in Morocco. *East Mediterr. Health J*. 10(4-5):474-481.

Campbell DI, Murch SH, Elia M, Sullivan PB, Sanyang MS, Jobarteh B, Lunn PG. 2003. Chronic T cell-mediated enteropathy in rural west African children: relationship with nutritional status and small bowel function. *Pediatr. Res.* 54(3):306-311.

Caulfield LE, De Onis M, Blossner M, Black RE. 2004. Undernutrition as an underlying cause of child deaths associated with diarrhea, pneumonia, malaria, and measles. *Am. J. Clin. Nutr*. 80(1), 193-198.

Chamberlin SL, Narins B, 2005. The Gale Encyclopedia of Neurological Disorders. Detroit, Thomson Gale. p. 1859-1870.

Chopra K, Kundu S, Chowdhury DS. 1989. Antibody response of infants in tropics to five doses of oral polio vaccine. *J. Trop. Pediatr*. 35(1):19-23.

Cobra C, Muhilal, Rusmil K, Rustama D, Djatnika, Suwardi SS, Permaesih D, Muherdiyantiningsih, Martuti S, Semba RD. 1997. Infant survival is improved by oral iodine supplementation. *J. Nutr.* 127(4):574-578.

D'Angio CT, Maniscalco WM, Pichichero ME. 1995. Immunologic response of extremely premature infants to tetanus, Haemophilus-influenzae, and polio immunizations. *Pediatrics*. 96(1 Pt 1):18-22.

Engell RE, Lim SS. 2013. Does clean water matter? An updated analysis of water supply and sanitation interventions and diarrhoeal diseases. *Lancet*. 381:544.

Gershwin ME, Nestel P, Keen CL, 2004. *Handbook of nutrition and immunity,* 1st ed. New York, Humana Pr Inc.

Ghendon YZ, Sanakoyeva II.1961. Comparison of the resistance of the intestinal tract to poliomyelitis virus (Sabin's strains) in persons after naturally and experimentally acquired immunity. *ActaVirol.* 5:265-273.

Goodman T, Dalmiya N, De Benoist B, Schultink W. 2000. Polio as a platform: Using national immunization days to deliver vitamin A supplements. *Bull. World Health Organ.* 78:305-314.

Grassly NC, Fraser C, Wenger J, Deshpande JM, Sutter RW, Heymann DL, Aylward RB. 2006. New strategies for the elimination of polio from India. *Science.* 314(5802):1150-1153.

Grassly NC, Jafari H, Bahl S, Durrani S, Wenger J, Sutter RW, et al. 2010. Asymptomatic wild-type poliovirus infection in India among children with previous oral poliovirus vaccination. *J. Infect. Dis.* 201(10):1535-1543.

Greenwood BM, Bradley-Moore AM, Bradley AK, Kirkwood BR, Gilles HM. 1986. The immune response to vaccination in undernourished and well-nourished Nigerian children. *Ann. Trop. Med. Parasitol.* 80(5):53 7-544.

Guerrant RL, DeBoer MD, Moore SR, Scharf RJ, Lima AA. 2013. The impoverished gut - a triple burden of diarrhoea, stunting and chronic disease. *Nat. Rev. Gastroenterol. Hepatol.* 10(4):220-229.

Habib MA, Soofi S, Sheraz A, Bhatti ZS, Okayasu H, Zaidi SZ, Molodecky NA, Pallansch MA, Sutter RW, Bhutta ZA. 2015. Zinc supplementation fails to increase the immunogenicity of oral poliovirus vaccine: a randomized controlled trial. *Vaccine.* 33(6):819-825.

Hagan JE, Wassilak SG, Craig AS, Tangermann RH, Diop OM, Burns CC, Quddus A; Centers for Disease Control and Prevention (CDC). 2015. Progress toward polio eradication - worldwide, 2014-2015. *MMWR Morb. Mortal Wkly Rep.* 64(19):527-531.

Hahn-Zoric M, Fulconis F, Minoli I, Moro G, Carlsson B, Böttiger M, Räihä N, Hanson LA. 1990. Antibody responses to parenteral and oral vaccines are impaired by conventional and low protein formulas as compared to breast-feeding. *Acta Paediatr. Scand.* 79(12):1137-1142.

Hamer D. 2010. Poliomyelitis. Public health and infectious diseases. 1st ed. Elsevier.

Handbook of resolutions and decisions of the World Health Assembly and the Executive Board. 3rd edition. III. Geneva: WHO 1993; 1985-1992. Resolution WHA. 41.28. *Global eradication of poliomyelitis by the year 2000.*

Haque R, Snider C, Liu Y, Ma JZ, Liu L, Nayak U, Mychaleckyj JC, Korpe P, Mondal D, Kabir M, Alam M, Pallansch M, Oberste MS, Weldon W, Kirkpatrick BD, Petri WA Jr. 2014. Oral polio vaccine response in breast fed infants with malnutrition and diarrhea. *Vaccine*. 32(4):478-482.

Hussain I, Mach O, Habib A, Bhatti Z, Suhag Z, Oberste MS, Weldon WC, Sutter RW, Soofi SB, Bhutta ZA. 2017. Seroprevalence of Anti-polio Antibodies in Children from Polio High-risk Areas of Pakistan: A Cross-Sectional Survey 2015-2016. *Pediatr. Infect. Dis. J.* 36(9):e230-e236.

Jafari H, Deshpande JM, Sutter RW, Bahl S, Verma H, Ahmad M, Kunwar A, Vishwakarma R, Agarwal A, Jain S, Estivariz C, Sethi R, Molodecky NA, Grassly NC, Pallansch MA, Chatterjee A, Aylward RB. 2014. Polio eradication. Efficacy of inactivated poliovirus vaccine in India. *Science*. 345(6199):922-925.

Jesmin A, Yamamoto SS, Malik AA, Haque MA. 2011. Prevalence and determinants of chronic malnutrition among preschool children: a cross-sectional study in Dhaka City, Bangladesh. *J. Health Popul. Nutr.* 29(5):494-499.

John TJ. 1975. Oral polio vaccination of children in the tropics. II. Antibody response in relation to vaccine virus infection. *Am. J. Epidemiol.* 102(5):414-421.

Kew OM, Cochi SL, Jafari HS, Wassilak SG, Mast EE, Diop OM, Tangermann RH, Armstrong GL; Centers for Disease Control and Prevention (CDC). 2014. Possible eradication of wild poliovirus type 3 -worldwide, 2012. *MMWR Morb. Mortal Wkly Rep*. 63(45):1031-1033.

Khare S, Kumari S, Nagpal IS, Sharma D, Verghese T. 1993. Oral polio vaccination in infants: beneficial effect of additional dose at birth. *Ind. J. Pediatr*. 60(2):275-281.

Korpe PS, Petri WA Jr. 2012. Environmental enteropathy: critical implications of a poorly understood condition. *Trends Mol. Med.* 18(6):328-336.

Langkamp DL, Langhough R. 1992. Primary care physicians' knowledge about diphtheria, tetanus and pertussis immunizations in preterm infants. *Pediatrics*. 8952-8955.

Langkamp DL, Langhough R. 1993. What do parents of preterm infants know about diphtheria, tetanus and pertussis immunizations? *Am. J. Perinatol.*10187-10189.

Lozano R, Naghavi M, Foreman K, Lim K, Shibuya K, Aboyans V, Abraham J, Adair T, Aggarwal R, Ahn SY, et al. 2012. Global and regional mortality from 235 causes of death for 20 age groups in 1990 and 2010: A systematic analysis for the Global Burden of Disease Study 2010. *Lancet*. 380:2095-2128.

Mahmood H. 2018. Polio Elimination in Pakistan: Still A Dream*? J. Ayub. Med. Coll. Abbottabad*. 30(2):304-307.

Martinez M, Shukla H, Ahmadzai M, Nikulin J, Wadood MZ, Ahmed J, Mbaeyi C, Jorba J, Ehrhardt D. 2018. Progress toward Poliomyelitis Eradication - Afghanistan, January 2017-May 2018. *MMWR Morb. Mortal Wkly Rep*. 67(30):833-837.

Moeti M. 2016. Winning the battle against the scourge of poliomyelitis in the African Region. *Vaccine*. 34(43):5142-5143.

Müller O., Krawinkel M. 2005. Malnutrition and health in developing countries. *Can. Med. Assoc. J.* 173:279-286.

Myaux JA, Unicomb L, Besser RE, Modlin JF, Uzma A, Islam AM, Santosham M. 1996. Effect of diarrhea on the humoral response to oral polio vaccination. *Pediatr. Infect. Dis. J.* 15(3):204-209.

Newton S, Cousens S, Owusu-Agyei S, Filteau S, Stanley C, Linsell L, Kirkwood B. 2005. Vitamin a supplementation does not affect infants' immune responses to polio and tetanus vaccines. *J. Nutr.* 135(11):2669-2673.

Okoko JB, Wesumperuma HL, Hart CA. 2001. The influence of prematurity and low birthweight on transplacental antibody transfer in a rural West African population. *Trop. Med. Int. Health*. 6(7):529-534.

O'Reilly KM, Durry E, ul Islam O, Quddus A, Abid N, Mir TP, Tangermann RH, Aylward RB, Grassly NC. 2012. The effect of mass immunisation campaigns and new oral poliovirus vaccines on the incidence of poliomyelitis in Pakistan and Afghanistan, 2001-11: a retrospective analysis. *Lancet*. 380(9840):491-498.

Patriarca PA, Wright PF, John TJ. 1991. Factors affecting the immunogenicity of oral poliovirus vaccine in developing countries: review. *Rev. Infect. Dis*. 13 (5):926-939.

Pickering LK, Granoff DM, Erickson JR, Masor ML, Cordle CT, Schaller JP, Winship TR, Paule CL, Hilty MD. 1998. Modulation of the immune system by human milk and infant formula containing nucleotides. *Pediatrics*. 101(2):242-249.

Rahman MM, Alvarez JO, Mahalanabis D, et al. 1997. Does simultaneous vitamin A supplementation with polio vaccine adversely affect seroconversion? XVIII Meeting of the International Vitamin A consultative Group, Cairo, Egypt, 1997 (poster).

Ross AC. 1992. Vitamin A status: relationship to immunity and the antibody response. *Proc. Soc. Exp. Biol. Med.* 200(3):303-320.

Saleem AF, Mach O, Quadri F, Khan A, Bhatti Z, Rehman NU, Zaidi S, Weldon WC, Oberste SM, Salama M, Sutter RW, Zaidi AK. 2015. Immunogenicity of poliovirus vaccines in chronically malnourished infants: a randomized controlled trial in Pakistan. *Vaccine*. 33(24):2757-2763.

Shah SZ, Saad M, RahmanKhattak MH, Rizwan M, Haidari A, Idrees F. 2016. "Why we could not eradicate polio from Pakistan and how can we?"*J. Ayub. Med. Coll. Abbottabad*. 28(2):423-425.

Sutter RW, Platt L, Mach O, Jafari H, Aylward RB. 2014. The new polio eradication end game: rationale and supporting evidence. *J. Infect. Dis.* 210 Suppl. 1:S434-S438.

Sutter RW, John TJ, Jain H, Agarkhedkar S, Ramanan PV, Verma H, Deshpande J, Singh AP, Sreevatsava M, Malankar P, Burton A, Chatterjee A, Jafari H, Aylward RB. 2010. Immunogenicity of bivalent types 1 and 3 oral poliovirus vaccine: a randomised, double-blind, controlled trial. *Lancet*. 376(9753):1682-1688.

Taffs RE, Enterline JC, Rusmil K, Muhilal, Suwardi SS, Rustama D, Djatnika, Cobra C, Semba RD, Cohen N, Asher DM. 1999. Oral iodine supplementation does not reduce neutralizing antibody responses to oral poliovirus vaccine. *Bull. World Health Organ.* 77(6):484-491.

Vohr BR, Oh W. 1986. Age of diphtheria, tetanus, and pertussis immunization of special care nursery graduates. *Pediatrics*. 77569-77571.

WHO independent monitoring board global polio eradication. 2013 May. 7th report.

WHO South-East Asia Region certified polio-free.WHO. Geneva; 27 March 2014. Available online at: http://www.searo.who.int/entity/campaigns/polio-certification/en/ accessed on 28 October 2018.

WHO Collaborative Study Group on Oral and Inactivated Poliovirus Vaccines. 1997. Combined immunization of infants with oral and inactivated poliovirus vaccines: results of a randomized trial in The Gambia, Oman, and Thailand. *J. Infect. Dis.* 175 Suppl. 1:S215-S227.

WHO. 2017. *Poliomyelitis.* In International travel and health. Available online at: http://www.who.int/ith/vaccines/polio/en/ accessed 26 June 2018.

World Health Organisation.2008. Progress towards interrupting wild poliovirus transmission worldwide, January 2007-April 2008. *WklyEpidemiol. Rec.* 83:170-176.

Wolf J, Prüss-Ustün A, Cumming O, Bartram J, Bonjour S, Cairncross S, Clasen T, Colford JM Jr, Curtis V, De France J, Fewtrell L, Freeman MC, Gordon B, Hunter PR, Jeandron A, Johnston RB, Mäusezahl D, Mathers C, Neira M, Higgins JP. 2014. Assessing the impact of drinking water and sanitation on diarrhoeal disease in low- and middle-income settings: systematic review and meta-regression. *Trop. Med. Int. Health.* 19(8):928-942.

Yousuf A, Syed Shah SA, Syed Jaffery IA, Ahmed SA, Khan MA, Aslam M. 2015. Seroprevalence rate of Poliovirus antibodies among the Healthy and Protein Energy Malnutrition children. *Pak. J. Med. Sci.* 31(2):403-407.

Zaman K, Sack DA, Yunus M, Arifeen SE, Podder G, Azim T, Luby S, Breiman RF, Neuzil K, Datta SK, Delem A, Suryakiran PV, Bock HL; Bangladeshi Rotavirus Vaccine study group. 2009. Successful co-administration of a human rotavirus and oral poliovirus vaccines in Bangladeshi infants in a 2-dose schedule at 12 and 16 weeks of age. *Vaccine*. 27(9):1333-1339.

In: Contemporary Issues in Childhood … ISBN: 978-1-53617-348-2
Editors: J. Ratan Ghosh and K. Bose

Chapter 4

A STUDY OF UNDERNUTRITION AMONG THE ADOLESCENT AHOM CHILDREN OF UPPER ASSAM

Dali Dutta and Sarthak Sengupta*
Department of Anthropology, Dibrugarh University, Dibrugarh, India

INTRODUCTION

The prevalence of undernutrition is considered to be major public health problem among the various population groups of India. The magnitude of undernutrition is observed to be greater among the most vulnerable segments of the population, especially in the rural regions. India shows the highest occurrence of childhood undernutrition in the World and it has been estimated that more than half of the Indian children are undernourished. The current nutritional status of children not only reflects their well being of the present time but also reflects future outcomes in terms of their health and development. Undernutrition is closely associated with a large proportion of child deaths (Seetharaman et al., 2007). Generally, three anthropometric indicators are often used to assess nutritional status during childhood: Weight for age used to measure low

*Corresponding Author's Email: sarthak@dibru.ac.in.

weight, also known as wasting, and height for age to measure stunting (slow skeletal growth) are two useful indices for assessing growth status and level of malnutrition of the children. For assessing malnutrition and evaluation of Protein-Calorie Malnutrition in growing children, the Body Mass Index is commonly used. Body Mass Index is recommended as the basis for anthropometric indicators of thinness and overweight during adolescence (Rolland Cachera, 1933).Growth during childhood is widely used to assess adequate health, nutrition, and development of children, and to estimate overall nutritional status as well as health status of a population. It is well documented that chronic undernutrition is associated with slower cognitive development and serious health impairment later in life which reduce the quality of life.

The present chapter is devoted to assess the nutritional status in terms of anthropometric characters of pre-adolescent and adolescent Ahom boys and girls of 6 to 15 years of age inhabiting in the rural areas of upper Assam.

The Ahom is one of the numerically dominant population of Assam. They are Mongoloid people. They belong to Tai-Mao or the Mao section of the Tai and are widely known as Shan. The Ahom people first came to India from Myanmar in 1228 A.D. and expanded their authority up to 1826 A.D. At present, Dhemaji, Dibrugarh, Lakhimpur, Sibsagar and Tinsukia district of upper Assam are the main concentration of the Ahom people.

MATERIAL AND METHODS

This community-basedcross-sectional study was conducted in a number of schools of the Lakhimpur, Sivsagar and Dibrugarh districts of Upper Assam. The study was carried out from January to December 2010. A total of 1172 children (boys= 563, girls= 609) aged 6-15 years were assessed. The children were further divided into two categories: pre-adolescent, i.e., 6-10 years and adolescents, i.e., 11-15 years of age. A total of 586 pre-adolescent children (282 boys and 304 girls) and 586 adolescents (281 boys and 305 girls) were measured and included in the present study. Anthropometric measurement of height and weight was done with a portable weighing machine and measuring scale, removing shoes and with minimal clothing. During measurement of weight and height norms of anthropometry were strictly followed. The first author (DD) herself recorded the anthropometric measurements. Children were considered underweight, stunting and thinness as weight-for-age, height-for-age, and body mass index for age Z-score below -2 standard deviation using the National Center for Health Statistics (NCHS) reference population. The present findings were compared with other available data from various population groups of Assam (Begum, 1995; Singh, 2008; Sikdar, 2010; Medhi, 2014; Deori, 2016).

The technical error measurement (TEM) was calculated following the method of Ulijaszek and Kerr (1999) and the coefficient of reliability (R) of the measurements was calculated to determine the reliability of the measurements. The intra-observed TEM were observed to be within the cut-off value of 0.95 as suggested by Ulijeszek and Kerr (1999). Hence, the measurements taken recorded in the present study were considered to be reliable and reproducible and the TEM values were not incorporated for further statistical consideration.The investigation was explained to all the students in their local language. The respondents, their guardian, as well as the school teacher were asked for their consent to participate and co-operate in the investigation in written form (in local vernacular).

RESULTS

The mean height and weight by age and sex were calculated and shown in Table 1. It is observed that significant sex difference existed in mean height at age 6, 14 and 15 years and in mean weight at age 6, 11-13 and 15 years. Moreover, there is increasing trends in mean height and weight in both sexes with advancement of age.

Table 2 shows that overall prevalence of underweight which is higher in boys having preponderance with moderate and severe (9.92% and 2.74% respectively) than the girls (7.53% and 2.57% respectively). It is apparent from the table that 27.66 percent pre-adolescent boys and 25.33 percent girls are in underweight category whereas 24.91 percent adolescent boys and only 13.44 percent girls are in underweight category. The adolescents Ahom children are thus in a better position than the pre-adolescents children.

The Ahom children were also analyzed for their height for expected age is shown in Table 3. It was found that 992 children were healthy while 180 children were stunted. Out of 180 stunted children, 80 (8.06%) were boys and 100 (10.08%) were girls. The analysis indicates that prevalence of stunting in girls is relatively higher than the boys' counterparts. Age wise stunting of children is also analyzed which shows that the onset of stunting is highest (2.74%) among the children of 6 years age group and lowest (0.68%) among the children of 11 years of age group. Most of the stunting girls are recorded in the adolescent period, i.e., 17.71 percent, whereas 11.75 percent adolescent boys are stunted. The pre-adolescent boys (16.67%) are more stunted than the preadolescent girls (15.13%).

Table 1. Mean values of anthropometric characteristics of the Ahom children according to age and sex

Age (in years)	Sex	Sample	Height	t value	Weight	t value
6	Male	67	109.68	2.53*	17.05	2.92*
	Female	57	107.28		15.91	
7	Male	53	119.66	1.53	20.33	0.58
	Female	60	117.96		19.98	
8	Male	54	123.26	1.35	21.42	1.68
	Female	54	121.83		20.53	
9	Male	55	129.30	0.55	24.73	0.74
	Female	64	128.70		24.20	
10	Male	53	131.49	0.21	25.74	0.27
	Female	69	131.72		25.93	
11	Male	54	137.71	1.63	28.51	3.49*
	Female	65	139.72		31.58	
12	Male	59	144.14	0.17	32.63	2.05*
	Female	70	144.36		34.66	
13	Male	53	148.73	0.68	36.18	2.03*
	Female	56	147.77		38.92	
14	Male	55	156.43	3.57*	41.78	0.55
	Female	51	151.29		42.49	
15	Male	60	163.65	8.99*	49.20	3.50*
	Female	63	152.32		44.27	

* indicates probability level <0.05.

Table 2. Prevalence of underweight among the Ahom children

Age in Years	Boys						Girls					
	≥-2 Z Score N %		-2 to -3 Z Score N %		≤-3 Z Score N %		≥-2 Z Score N %		-2 to -3 Z Score N %		≤-3 Z Score N %	
6	40	59.70	20	29.85	7	10.45	31	54.39	14	24.56	12	21.05
7	43	81.13	5	9.43	5	9.43	51	85.00	7	11.67	2	3.33
8	39	72.22	13	24.07	2	3.70	40	74.07	9	16.67	5	9.26
9	43	78.18	10	18.18	2	3.64	53	82.81	10	15.63	1	1.56
10	39	73.58	10	18.87	4	7.55	52	75.36	12	17.39	5	7.25
6-10	204	72.34	58	20.57	20	7.09	227	74.67	52	17.11	25	8.22
	$X^2 = 1.29$, d. f = 2											
11	42	77.78	12	22.22	-		54	83.08	10	15.38	1	1.54
12	42	71.19	15	25.42	2	3.39	61	87.14	7	10.00	2	2.86
13	35	66.04	15	28.30	3	5.66	49	87.50	5	8.93	2	3.57
14	41	74.55	8	14.55	6	10.91	47	92.16	4	7.84	-	
15	51	85.00	8	13.33	1	1.67	53	84.13	10	15.87	-	
11-15	211	75.09	58	20.64	12	4.27	264	86.56	36	11.80	5	1.64
	$X^2 = 12.99^*$, d. f = 2											
6-15	415	35.50	116	9.92	32	2.74	491	42.00	88	7.53	30	2.57

* indicates probability level <0.05; ≥-2 Z score = Normal, -2 to -3 Z score = Moderate, <-3 Z score = Severe underweight.

Prevalence of thinness categories as based on the WHO cut-offs is shown in Table 4. WHO cut-offs were determined using LMS method. It is reveals from the table that the overall prevalence of thinness is comparatively higher among Ahom boys (13.34%) than the Ahom girls (7.10%). The prevalence of thinness is more among the pre-adolescent children (32.98% boys and 23.03% girls) than adolescent children (22.42% boys and 4.26% girls) respectively.

According to WHO (1995) classification of severity in malnutrition, the overall prevalence of underweight is high (20.0-29.0%). However, the prevalence of stunting was low (<20.0%).

Table 5 shows the comparison of nutritional status of Ahom with other population groups of Assam. The frequency of underweight in Ahom boys (12.66%) is higher than the Deori (7.94%) population. On the other hand, the frequency is much less than the Sonowal Kachari (23.12%), Mishing (30.10%), Assamese Muslim (46.95%), and Bengali Muslim (51.45%). The

Ahom girls also record more underweight (10.10%) than the Deori (2.51%) girls. However, they are having less underweight than the Sonowal Kachari (16.13%), Mishing (33.30%), Assamese Muslim (47.74%) and Bengali Muslim (52.87%).

The frequency of stunted Ahom boys (6.84%) is far less than Sonowal Kachari (17.41%), Assamese Muslim (20.56%), Deori (28.26%), Mishing (28.90%) and Bengali Muslim (41.48%). The incidence of stunted Ahom girls (8.55%) is also comparatively less than the Assamese Muslim (21.11%), Sonowal Kachari (23.32%), Deori (28.25%), Mishing (33.30%) and Bengali Muslim (43.95%). Thus, it is apparent that both girls and boys are less stunted than the other population groups of Assam.

With respect to prevalence of thinness cases, it is seen that the Ahom boys are more in number in thinness category (13.34%) than the Deori (8.67%) and Sonowal Kachari (10.13%) boys.

Table 3. Prevalence of stunting among the Ahom children

Age in years	≥-2 Z Score N %		-2 to -3 Z Score N %		≤-3 Z Score N %		≥-2 Z Score N %		-2 to -3 Z Score N %		≤-3 Z Score N %	
6	53	79.10	11	16.42	3	4.47	39	68.42	13	22.81	5	8.77
7	43	81.13	9	16.98	1	1.89	54	90.00	5	8.33	1	1.67
8	44	81.48	8	14.81	2	3.70	45	83.33	9	16.67	-	
9	50	90.91	5	9.09	-		60	93.75	4	6.25	-	
10	45	84.91	8	15.09			60	86.96	9	13.04	-	
6-10	235	83.33	41	14.54	6	2.13	258	84.87	40	13.16	6	1.97
	$X^2 = 0.26$, d. f = 2											
11	52	96.27	2	3.70	-		59	90.77	4	6.15	2	3.08
12	53	89.83	6	10.17	-		58	82.86	10	14.29	2	2.86
13	44	83.02	9	16.98	-		45	80.36	9	16.07	2	3.57
14	44	80.00	9	16.36	2	3.64	45	88.24	6	11.76	-	
15	55	91.67	4	6.67	1	1.67	44	69.84	18	28.57	1	1.59
11-15	248	88.26	30	10.68	3	1.07	251	82.30	47	15.41	7	2.30
	$X^2 = 4.40$, d. f = 2											
6-15	483	41.32	71	6.07	9	0.77	509	43.54	87	7.44	13	1.11

Note: * indicates probability level < 0.05; ≥-2 Z score = Normal; -2 to -3 Z score = Moderate; <-3 Z score = Severely stunted.

Table 4. Prevalence of thinness among the Ahom children

Age in Years	Boys						Girls					
	≥-2 Z Score N %		-2 to -3 Z Score N %		≤-3 Z Score N %		≥-2 Z Score N %		-2 to -3 Z Score N %		≤-3 Z Score N %	
6	40	59.70	15	22.39	12	17.91	38	66.67	10	17.54	9	15.79
7	34	64.15	11	20.75	8	15.09	48	80.00	10	16.67	2	3.33
8	34	62.96	15	27.78	5	9.26	40	74.07	9	16.67	5	9.26
9	40	72.73	10	18.18	5	9.09	53	82.81	9	14.06	2	3.13
10	41	77.36	8	15.09	4	7.55	55	79.71	13	18.84	1	1.45
6-10	189	67.02	59	20.92	34	12.06	234	76.97	51	16.78	19	6.25
	$X^2 = 8.79^*$, d.f = 2											
11	42	77.78	12	22.22	-		61	93.85	3	4.62	1	1.54
12	43	72.88	12	20.34	4	6.78	65	92.86	3	4.29	2	2.86
13	37	69.81	12	22.64	4	7.55	55	98.21	1	1.79		
14	44	80.00	8	14.55	3	5.45	50	98.04	1	1.96		
15	52	86.67	7	11.67	1	1.67	61	96.83	2	3.17		
11-15	218	77.58	51	18.15	12	4.27	292	95.74	10	3.28	3	0.98
	$X^2 = 42.78^*$, d. f = 2											
6-15	407	34.82	110	9.41	46	3.93	526	44.99	61	5.22	22	1.88

Note: * indicates probability level <0.05; ≥-2 Z score = Normal; -2 to -3 Z score = Moderate; ≤-3 Z score = Severely thinness.

Table 5. Nutritional status of Ahom and other population groups of Assam

Population	Underweight (%)		Stunted (%)		Low BMI for age (%)		Source
	Boys	Girls	Boys	Girls	Boys	Girls	
Ahom	12.66	10.10	6.84	8.55	13.34	7.10	Present Study
Deori	7.94	2.51	28.26	28.25	8.67	6.81	Deori, 2016
Sonowal Kachari	23.12	16.13	17.41	23.32	10.13	6.10	Singh, 2008
Mishing	30.10	33.30	28.90	33.30	20.70	18.00	Sikdar, 2010
Assamese Muslim	46.95	47.74	20.56	21.11	65.48	68.59	Begum, 1995
Bengali Muslim	51.45	52.87	41.48	43.95	51.12	53.50	Medhi, 2014

However, a case of thinness is much less than the Mishing (20.70%), Assamese Muslim (65.48%) and Bengali Muslim (51.12%). In case of the girls, 7.10 percent of Ahom girls are in thinness category whereas only 6.10 percent of the Sonowal Kachari, 6.81 percent of Deori girls belongs to thinness category. Incidence of thinness is considerably high among the

Mishing (18.00%), Assamese Muslim (68.59%) and Bengali Muslim (53.50%) than the Ahom girls.

DISCUSSION

The present investigation is based on the WHO proposed cut-offs given for the assessment of undernutrition among pre-adolescents and adolescents in terms of underweight, stunting, and thinness. Present study shows that 11.75 percent of boys and 17.71 percent of adolescent girls are in stunting category. Findings of the study conducted by Medhi et al. (2006) contradict our results who recorded as high as 50.1 percent of boys and 43.1 percent of girls from Assam suffered from stunting. Similarly, overall prevalence of stunting in the present Ahom sample is 29.46 percent among adolescents, however, Mondal and Terangpi (2014) recorded 51.2 percent of Karbi adolescents are stunted. Thinness among the Ahom children is 26.68 percent as against only 13.4 percent of thinness recorded among Karbi adolescents (ibid, 2014).

CONCLUSION

Overall (age and sex combined) prevalence of underweight (severe + moderate), stunting and thinness is 22.75 percent, 15.40 percent, and 20.44 percent, respectively. Of these, 5.30 percent, 1.88 percent, and 5.82 percent of Ahom children were found to be severely underweight, stunted and thinness respectively. Present study shows that Ahom children of both sexes are facing a risk in terms of nutritional status (e.g., underweight). The study also records that the prevalence of underweight among the Ahom children of Assam is more than the incidence of stunting and thinness. It also demonstrates that the children, as well as adolescents of the community, relatively show better nutritional status than the other neighbouring population groups. However, the community needs appropriate support for proper implementation of health and nutritional programmes so that their nutritional status can be better managed.

REFERENCES

Begum, G 1995, *Age Changes in Some Somatometric Characters with Reference to Nutritional Status of Assamese Muslims of Kamrup District,* Assam. PhD Thesis, Gauhati University.

Deori, J 2016, *A Cross-Sectional Study on Physical Growth among the Deoris of Assam and Arunachal Pradesh.* PhD Thesis, Gauhati University.

Medhi, D 2013, *Growth, and Nutritional Status among the Muslims of Barpeta District Assam.* Ph D Thesis, Gauhati University.

Medhi, G K, Barua, A and Mahanta, J 2006, 'Growth and nutritional status of school-age children (6-14Years) of tea garden workers of Assam,' *Journal of Human Ecology*, vol. 19, no.2, pp. 83-85.

Mondal, N, and Moloya, T 2014, 'Prevalence of undernutrition among tribal adolescents of Karbi Anglong district of Assam, Northeast India,'*Sri Lanka Journal of Child Health*, vol.43, no.3, pp. 154-157.

National Centre for Health Statistics (N.C.H.S), 2000, CDC Growth Charts for the United States: Methods and Development. *Series Report* 11, No. 241.

Rolland-Cachera, MF 1933, 'Body composition during adolescence: Methods, limitations and determinants,' *Hormonal Research* (Suppl.), vol.39, pp. 55-66.

Seetharaman, N, Chacko, TV, Shankar SRL, Mathew, AC 2007, 'Measuring malnutrition, the role of Z scores and the composite index of Anthropometric failure (CIAF).' *Indian J. Comm.Med.*, vol.32, pp. 35-39.

Sikdar, M 2010, *Bio Social Determinants of Growth and Nutritional Status of the Mishings of Upper Assam.* PhD Thesis, Dibrugarh University, Dibrugarh.

Singh, J 2008, *A Study on Growth and Nutritional Status of the Sonowal Kachari of Dibrugarh District*, Assam. PhD Thesis, Dibrugarh University, Dibrugarh.

Ulijaszek, SJ and Kerr, DA 1999, 'Anthropometric measurement error and the assessment of nutritional status,' *British Journal of Nutrition*, vol.82, pp.165-177.

World Health Organization. 1995. *Physical Status: The Use and Interpretation of Anthropometry*. Technical Report Series No. 854. Geneva: World Health Organization.

In: Contemporary Issues in Childhood … ISBN: 978-1-53617-348-2
Editors: J. Ratan Ghosh and K. Bose

Chapter 5

Fat Free Mass and Fat Mass in Indian Infants: Relevance of 'Thin-Fat' Phenotype

Dilip Mahalanabis and Bandana Sen*
Society for Applied studies, Salt Lake City, Kolkata, West Bengal, India

Abstract

Obesity and under nutrition represent the two extremes on the spectrum of adiposity in infants and children and pose a major health problem globally. Adult cardiovascular disease, type 2 diabetes and metabolic syndrome are increased in people who were light and thin at birth and during infancy. Adiposity is routinely quantified in terms of weight and height relative to the child's age. Body mass index (BMI) is widely used to indicate adiposity in adults and recently also in children. However, anthropometry is inadequate to distinguish fat mass (FM) from fat free mass (FFM). Babies in South Asia have lower birth weight than in the West; their body-fat is relatively preserved leading to their description as 'thin-fat'.

*Corresponding Author's Email: sascf198@yahoo.com.

Their relatively higher percentage of body fat (FM%) at birth was shown to track through childhood to adulthood.

Recently we have developed two sets of validated equations to predict FFM and FM, one based on skinfold thicknesses and mid arm circumference and the other on bioelectrical impedance analysis (BIA). For both sets we used D_2O dilution as reference method.

Using the newly developed BIA equations on 331 infants and children aged 6m to 24m of age the mean (SD) FM% was 15.36 (5.34). Using the equations based on skinfold thicknesses and mid arm circumference the mean (SD) FM% in the same 331 children was 17.01 (6.05). Among 55 (17%) of the 331 children who had weight for height Z-score of -2 or less (i.e., lean) 6 (11%) had FM of 20% or more by the skinfold/mid arm circumference based equations and 5(9%) by BIA equations. About 10% of the lean children had relatively high FM% whom we consider to be 'thin fat' phenotype as described above.

To conclude, we developed and validated new improved tools to measure adiposity in infants and young children suitable for South Asia. We applied these equations on a group of children 6m to 24m from among the urban low-middle class families in India. In a proportion of them (10%) the FM% was relatively retained in spite of leanness i.e., weight for height Z-score $\leq$-2 and are considered to be 'thin-fat' phenotype.

VALIDATION OF PUBLISHED EQUATIONS

Techniques for validation such as underwater weighing are not feasible in infants and young children. Use of methods that involve any degree of radiation (e.g., DEXA, radioactive tracers) is also not desirable for infants. We therefore used a stable isotope dilution technique as the reference standard.

Eighty-six children participated in the present deuterium oxide (D_2O) study. In eight of them, the D_2O procedures were incomplete because of vomiting or being fed during the equilibration period. They were dropped from the study. The study infants were predominantly breast-fed (88%). The D_2O procedures were completed in 78 children. We validated the 5 published equations two based on anthropometry (Mellits& Cheek, 1970 (AN-1) & Morgenstern et al., 2002 (AN-2)) and three based on BIA (Fjeld et al., 1990 (BI1), Bocage, 1988 (BI2) & Kushner et al,. 1992 (BI3)) on 52 children for FFM and FM in kg using the reference method D_2O dilution technique (Sen at al., 2008, 2010). Mean FFM derived by all the five methods were comparatively lower than the ones by the reference method (Table 1). Mean FFM derived by AN-1 was 2.22% lower than the reference method ($p=0.002$) and FFM derived by AN-2 was 0.68% lower than D_2O dilution ($p=0.29$). The mean FFM values derived by BI1, BI2, and BI3 were 2.76% ($p=0.003$), 5.49% ($p<0.001$) and 11.5% ($p<0.001$) lower than the reference method respectively.

Table 1. The mean and SD of FFMkg and as % body weight derived by the five equations under study and by the D_2O dilution technique (Reference method)

Methods	FFMkg: Mean ± SD (%FFM: Mean ± SD)
D_2O dilution	7.28 ± 1.13 (82.56 ± 7.59)
Anthropometry (AN-1)	7.11 ± 1.09 (80.35 ± 2.46)
Anthropometry (AN-2)	7.25 ± 1.13 (81.88 ± 3.66)
BIA (BI1)	7.05 ± 0.98 (79.80 ± 2.50)
BIA (BI2)	6.83 ±1.13 (77.07 ± 3.26)
BIA (BI3)	6.29 ± 1.10 (71.02 ± 5.77)

Similarly, FM derived by AN-1, AN-2, BI1, BI2 and BI3 were 2.22%, 0.68%, 2.76%, 5.49% and 11.5% higher than the reference method respectively. As expected, the mean FFM in boys tended to be higher than that in the girls for all Anthropometry and BIA methods. The differences however did not reach statistical significance. The mean and standard deviations of paired values of the difference in FFM in kg and as percentage of body weight between those derived by D_2O dilution and each of the three equations under study and 95% CI of the difference are shown in Table 2.

Table 2. The Mean, SD of the difference in FFM (of paired values) in kg and as percent of body weight between those derived by D_2O dilution and by each of the five equations under study and 95% confidence interval of the difference

	Mean difference in kg, (as % body weight)	SD	95% CI	P*
[a]D_2O-AN-1	0.18 (2.30)	0.57 (6.39	0.05 to 0.31 (0.89 to 3.74)	0.007 (0.002)
[b]D_2O-AN-2	0.04 (0.80)	0.57 (6.51)	-0.09 to 0.17 (-0.67 to 2.26)	0.50 (0.29)
[c]D_2O-BI1	0.25 (2.98)	0.56 (6.29)	0.13 to 0.38 (1.57 to 4.40)	0.002 (0.001)
[d]D_2O-BI2	0.47 (5.72)	0.57 (6.60)	0.34 to 0.60 (4.23 to 7.21)	<0.001 (<0.001)
[e]D_2O-BI3	1.41 (16.25)	0.60 (7.18)	1.28 to 1.55 (14.63 to 17.87)	<0.001 (<0.001)

[a]difference between D_2O method and Anthropometry methods of Mellits& Cheek 1970
[b]difference between D_2O method and Anthropometry methods of Morgenstern 2002
[c]difference between D_2O method and Bioelectrical Impedance analysis of Fjeld et al. 1990
[d]difference between D_2O method and Bioelectrical Impedance analysis of Bocage 1988)
[e]difference between D_2O method and Bioelectrical Impedance analysis of Kushner et al. 1992
*The t-test evaluates the difference of the paired values from zero.

Distribution of points for FFMkg along the line of identity (i.e., at 45^0) between D_2O and each of AN-1, AN-2, BI1, BI2 and BI3 method respectively, are shown in Figure 1(a)-(e). Bland- Altman plots of the differences of FFMkg in each participant between D_2O and each of the equations AN-1, AN-2, BI1, BI2 and BI3 against average FFMkg are shown Figure 2(f)-(j); mean differences were 0.18, 0.04, 0.25, 0.47, 1.41 respectively were shown.

For comparison of all these anthropometry and BIA methods, the results showed that the FFMkg derived by the equation of AN-2 and BI1 gives a better agreement with the reference method; 95% limits of agreement with the reference method (i.e., mean ± 2SD) were -0.81 to 1.11 and -0.91 to 1.01 for AN-1 and AN-2; -0.74 to 1.14, -0.55 to 1.29 and -0.16 to 1.76 for BI1, BI2 and BI3 respectively.

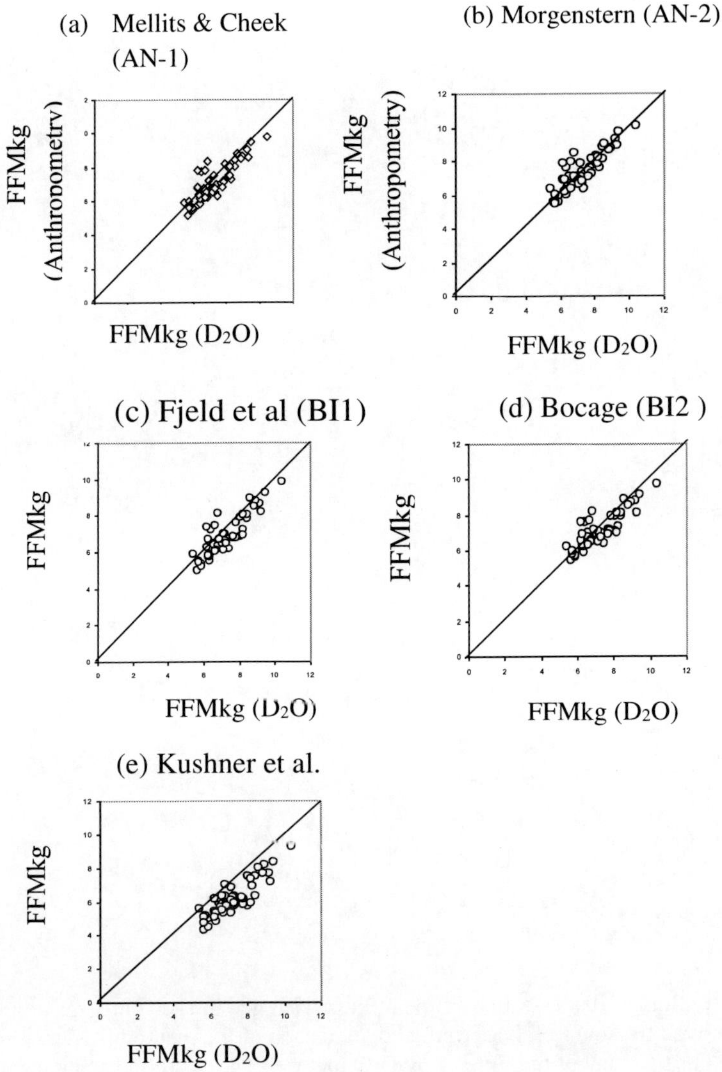

Figure 1. (a,b,c,d,e): FFMkg: Individual data points comparing values derived by the reference method (D_2O dilution) with those by the five equations under study are plotted along the "line of identity" (at 45^0angle). ANTHFFMkg: FFMkg derived by the two equations based on anthropometry (AN-1 & AN-2), plotted against D_2O method (R^2=0.75, R^2=0.76 respectively). BIAFFMkg: FFMkg derived by the three equations based on Bio electrical Impedance Analysis (BI1, BI2 &BI3) plotted against (R^2=0.74, R^2=0.76 & R^2=0.73 respectively). D_2OFFM kg: FFMkg derived by D_2O dilution method.

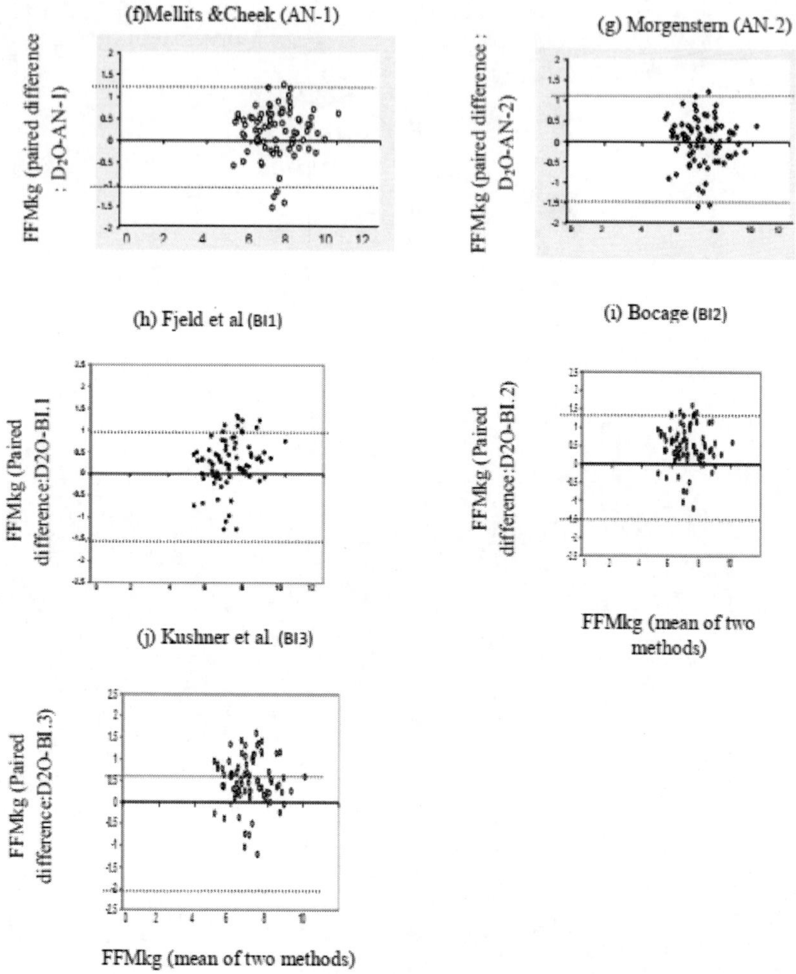

Figure 2. (f,g,h,i,j): Bland –Altman plots of the difference in each participant between FFMkg derived by D_2O as reference method and each of the methods under study plotted against average of the FFMkg by D_2O method. The solid line and the dotted lines are the mean and 2 SD are the mean and 2SD of the differences, respectively.

D_2O-AN-1: mean difference = 0.18, SD= 0.57, p=0.007.

D_2O-AN-2: mean difference = 0.04, SD= 0.57, p=0.505.

D_2O-BI1: mean difference = 0.25, SD= 0.56, p=0.0002.

D_2O-BI2: mean difference = 0.47, SD= 0.57, p<0.0001.

D_2O-BI3: mean difference = 1.04, SD= 0.59, p<0.0001.

We showed that the percentage of FFM in Indian infants derived by all the three method were consistently higher than the reference values in the US infants, indicating that the Indian infants are considerably leaner and have lower FM percentage.

Individual data points for percentage of FFM derived by the BIA equation of Fjeld et al., 1990 and by the reference method are plotted against age in months. Age and sex specific reference data on percentage FFM in healthy American infants derived by multicomponent models are also plotted for comparison. As expected, the percentage of FFM was consistently higher than the reference values for healthy infants from the USA (Figure 3).

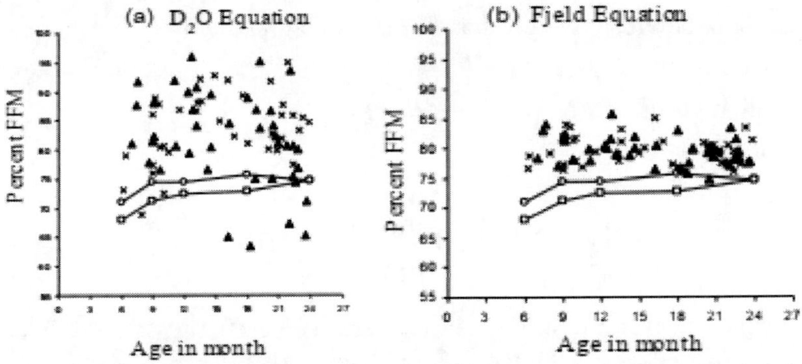

Figure 3. Individual data points for percentage of fat-free mass (FFM) derived by D_2O dilution method (a) and the bioelectrical impedance analysis equation of Fjeld et al,1990 (b) are plotted against age in months. Age and sex-specific reference values for percentage of FFM in healthy American infants derived by multicomponent models (Butte et al., 2000) are plotted for comparison (data points are connected). Boys(×), Girls(▲), boys(-○- ,Butte NF) girls(-□- ,Butte NF).

DEVELOPMENT OF NEW EQUATIONS

The best fit equations derived by regression models were first examined on the infants on whom the equations were developed. We used them on a new set of infants in the same age group who also had D_2O dilution test and compared the %body fat derived by the developed equations and by D_2O reference method. Percent fat derived by the new equations were plotted against those based on the equation for D_2O dilution by scatter diagrams and agreement was visually examined to note if the points lie close to the "line of equality" (i.e., the line at a 45^0 angle). Further more, the difference in %body fat for each child of the validation set between those derived by the new equations and by D_2O dilution was evaluated for their difference from zero by t-test. For reasonably symmetric distribution we expect the range, mean ± 2SD, to include about 95% of the observations and we used this to indicate 95% limits of agreement (Altman DJ, 1992). To evaluate how well the methods are likely to agree for comparing groups, we used 95% confidence interval of the mean of the differences in each subject to examine the agreement between two groups. For a good agreement we expect that the range, mean of the difference ± 2SE, to indicate 95% limits of agreement within which group means will lie 95% of the time.

Regression Equations

Multiple linear regression analyses were applied to the data to select the combination of variables which would give the lowest Root Mean Square Error (RMSE) and highest adjusted R^2. Initially higher order polynomial terms were included in a regression to test for nonlinearity. This was done univariately for each independent variable with FFMkg derived by D_2O dilution method as the dependant variable. For developing the equations, we have added one variable at a time as predictor variables as stated earlier and examined the values of adjusted R^2. The adjusted R^2 values are shown for each model with increasing number of predictor variables. In this way, the last model (i.e., model 5) was the best fit for girls and for boys model 2 was the best fit model. Model 5 included biceps, MAC (Mid Arm Circumference), age^2, and $triceps^2$ and model 2 included biceps and suprailiac as predictor variables. We have taken these values to construct the final equations, which are (Sen et al., 2010).

Girls: %body fat= $-69.26 + 5.76 \times B - 0.33 \times T^2 + 5.40 \times M + 0.01 \times A^2$ (1)

Boys: %body fat= $-8.75 + 3.73 \times B + 2.57 \times S$ (2)

where B = biceps skinfold thickness in mm, T = triceps skinfold thickness in mm, S = suprailiac skinfold thickness in mm, M = mid arm circumference in cm, and A = age in month.

In the same way, using regression models, we developed a BIA based equations for FFM in kg (FFMkg) (Sen et al., 2017).

FFMkg $=0.72+0.30*(\text{weight})+0.16*(\text{sex})+0.52*(\text{Length}^2/\text{resistance})$ (3)

where, Length in cm, Weight in kg, Resistance in Ω, sex: (Boys=1, Girls=0).

Evaluation Using New Skinfold Thickness Equation as Stated Earlier

The mean (SD) of the FM% calculated by the new equations were 17.11 (6.25) and 16.93 (6.02) for girls and boys respectively. Likewise mean (SD) of %body fat calculated by D_2O dilution methods were 17.11 (7.25) and 16.93 (6.62) for girls and boys respectively. The 95% confidence limits of the mean of the difference in %body fat derived by D_2O and by the new equations were -1.45 to +1.45 percent for girls and -1.33 to +1.33 percent for boys. As expected, the mean of the difference in %body fat was zero.

Bioelectrical Impedance Analysis

BIA measures impedance of the body to a small electric current. The generic theoretical model treats the body as a single cylinder, with measurements made between electrodes placed manually on the wrist and ankle. Adjustment of bioelectrical data for height allows estimation of TBW. The theoretical relation (Nyboer,0 1972) is as follows:

$$V \alpha L^2/Z$$

where V is the volume of the body water in the subject, Z is impedance, and L is the length of the subject. In our study, impedance and resistance were measured with a multi-frequency bioelectrical impedance analyzer (Xitron model 4000b; Xitrons technologies Inc. San Diego, USA) using a single frequency of 50 kHz. Children with dry light clothes lay supine (Deurenberg et al. 1989, 1988) with arms apart from the body and legs separated so that the thighs did not touch. After cleaning the skin contact area with alcohol, one pair of electrodes (foil disposable 5 cm^2 ECG electrodes) was placed on the dorsal surfaces of the right hand at the distal metacarpal joints and between the distal prominence of the right radius and ulna. Another pair was placed at the distal metatarsal joints and between the lateral malleoli of the right foot. The BIA is a simple and eminently suitable method as an epidemiological tool and is the only practical method that estimates FFM and this newly developed prediction equation should be suitable for this population.

Applicability of the Predictive Equations

Using the new prediction equations (1 and 2) we calculated the percent fat in an independent sample of 23 infants (11 girls and 12 boys) in the same age group and from the same community; we also calculated %body fat on them using the D_2O dilution equation. Mean (SD) of the predicted %body fat derived by the new skinfold thickness equations were 20.15 (7.06) and 14.21 (4.27) and by the D_2O dilution were 19.22 (9.54) and 15.36 (4.49) for girls and boys respectively. The mean (SE) of the difference in %body fat of the new skinfold and D_2O methods were -0.93 (1.98) for girls and 1.14 (0.70) for boys. The mean (SD) for the difference in %body fat were -0.93 (6.56) percent for girls and 1.14 (2.43) percent for boys. Distribution of data points along the line of identity (45^0) between %body fat derived from D_2O dilution method and by the new equation applied on the validated group have shown in Figure 4(a). The Bland-Altman, 1990 plots of the paired differences between the %body fat derived by D_2O reference method and the new equations for the validation group of girls and boys are plotted against average %body fat derived by D_2O method and respective new equations (Figure 4(b)).

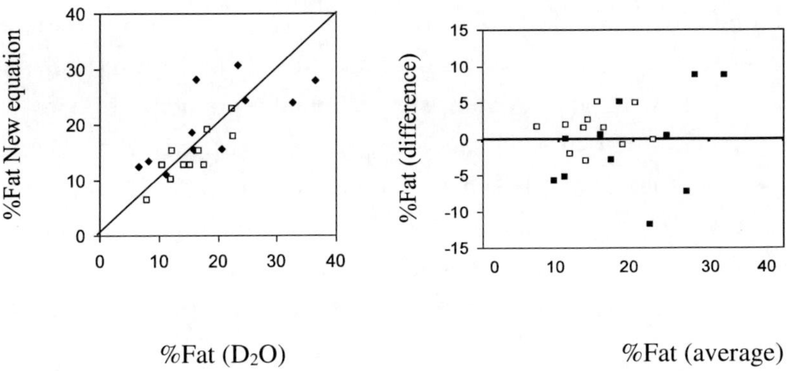

(a) (b)

Figure 4. (a): Individual data points of percent body fat (%fat) comparing values derived by the reference method (D_2O dilution) with the new predictive equations for Validation group of girls (▪) and boys (▫) under study along the "line of identity" (at 45^0angle). (b): Bland –Altman plots of the difference between %fat derived by D_2O reference method and the new equations for validation group of girls (▪) and for boys (▫) plotted against average %fat derived by D_2O method and respective new equation.

[a:] mean difference = -0.93, SD= 6.56.
[b:] mean difference = 1.14, SD= 2.43.

Application of the New BIA Equation

We calculated the body composition in an independent sample of 328 infants and children (164 boys and 164 girls) of similar age group and from the same community. We used the total fat free mass (FFM) and fat mass

(FM) derived from the weight and FFM to separate BMI into a fat mass index (FMI) and a fat free mass index (FFMI) as described by Demerath EW et al., 2006

$$BMI = Weight/height^2 = FM/height^2 + FFM/height^2 = FMI + FFMI$$
(Weight, FM and FFM are in kg, height in meters).

In a two component model body composition may be expressed as FMI and FFMI as earlier suggested by Van Itallie and colleagues (Van Itallie et al., 1990). In developed countries, BMI values steadily fall after the age of 1 year to a minimum around 6 years of age (on average) when it starts to increase and this phenomenon has been termed adiposity rebound (Rolland-Chachera et al., 1987), and age of adiposity rebound is predictive of obesity. In a longitudinal study of a large cohort of neonates Eriksson JG and colleagues (Eriksson et al., 2003) have shown that early adiposity rebound is associated with obesity in childhood and adult life and higher cumulative incidence of type 2 diabetes. In our larger sample of infants and young children, we notice a trend for adiposity rebound at an early age of 12-15 months (Figure 5).

BMI was split into FMI and FFMI for this larger sample and plotted against age in month (Figure 6). The FFMI trajectories in the study children do not follow the pattern of BMI in that there is no discernable rebound around 12-15 months of age. On the other hand the FMI showed a distinct adiposity rebound around the same age as seen for BMI trajectory suggesting that adiposity rebound is indeed associated with FMI trajectory. The study children are generally lean as reflected in the very low FMI compared to reference children. Maynard LM and colleagues (Maynard et al., 2001) have shown that the average incremental changes in BMI in children are associated with marked variability in body composition changes depending on the sex and age. In a study in older children aged 8 to 18 years Demerath EW and Colleagues (Demerath et al., 2006) have shown a curvilinear (J shaped) relationship between BMI percentile and FM% (Figure 7). Fat mass per unit of fat free mass is a better indicator if fatness (Figure 8). Their study indicates that BMI in children in the overweight ranges shows an association with higher adiposity compared to those in low to middle weight range. We plotted the FMI and FFMI in these study children against BMI values (Figure-9). These infants and young children show a similar trend i.e., higher BMI is associated with increasing FMI while FFMI shows a near linear relationship.

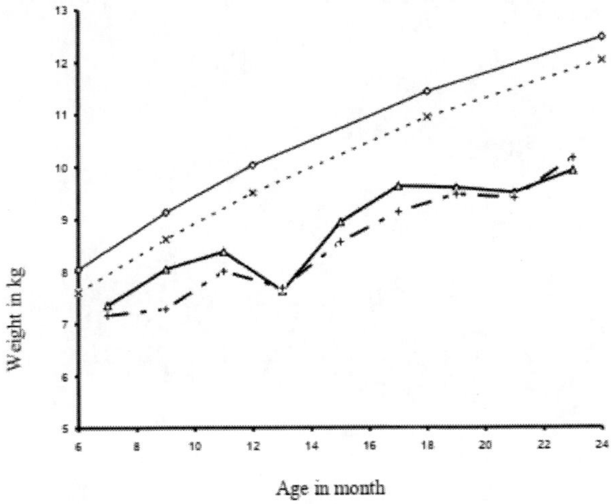

Figure 5. Age in month (average of 2 monthly data points) versus Weight in kg in study children compared to reference children (Butte et al., 2000). —□—reference Boy; ---x-- reference Girl; —Δ— Study boy; ---o---- Study girl.

Some characteristics of these 328 infants and children raise concern. They come from a low- middle socio economic strata in a metropolitan city in India and they represent a large urban population. The average birth weight in India is low (Sen et al., 2005, Gurav et al., 2003, Muthayya et al., 2009) and the proportion underweight (i.e., <2500 g) at birth is as high as 28% (Unicef, 2012). Body weight and BMI trajectory during 6 m-12 m indicate poor growth during infancy. Further they show a trend for very early adiposity rebound. These 3 factors i.e., LBW, poor weight gain in infancy and a likelihood of early adiposity rebound make such children vulnerable to chronic adult diseases (like CHD, type 2 diabetes, hypertension, stroke and osteoporosis) (Eriksson et al., 1999, Osmond et al., 1993, Frankel et al., 1996, Rich Edward et al., 1976, Eriksson et al., 2001, Barker, 2001). High rates of CHD and type 2 diabetes are being reported by the developing countries in one or two generations (Bulatao et al., 1992, Fall, 2001) and the predicted epidemics of them are expected to intensify, particularly in India over the next two decades (Wild et al., 2004). It is therefore of considerable interest to study the body composition in infants and children to better understand the phenomenon of the developmental origin of chronic adult diseases and this new equation should provide a useful tool for population based studies.

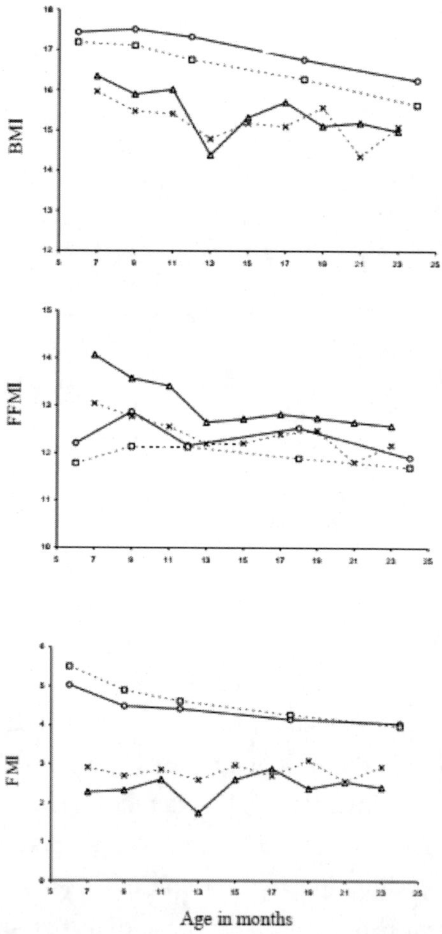

Figure 6. BMI, FFMI and FMI (average of two monthly data points) of the study children (n=328) plotted against age in month. For comparison we have plotted the age specific reference data on infants and children in USA derived by multicomponent modeling (Butte et al. 2000). —o— Reference (Boys), --□---- Reference (Girls), —Δ— study Boys and --×-- study girls.

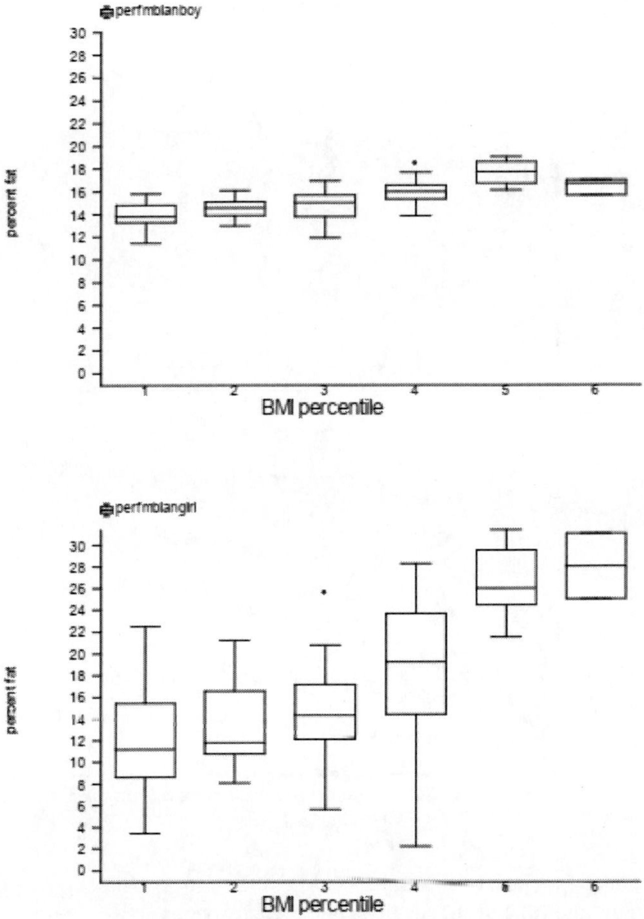

Figure 7. Box plots of FM% derived by BIA based (Fjeld et al., 1990) equations by body mass index percentile (BMIP) groups in boys (a) and girls (b) are shown. The BMIP groups are, BMIP≤5 =1(boys: 45, girls: 25), BMIP>5 &≤10 = 2 (boys: 10, girls: 16), BMIP>10 &≤25= 3 (boys: 34, girls: 38), BMIP>25 &≤85 = 4 (boys: 52, girls: 56), BMIP>85 &≤94 = 5 (boys: 8, girls: 5), and BMIP≥94 =6 (boys: 3, girls: 2). The line in the middle of the box represents the median. The box extends from the 25th percentile to 75th percentile. The lines emerging from the box are upper or lower adjacent rules which extend ± 1.5 times the interquartile range.

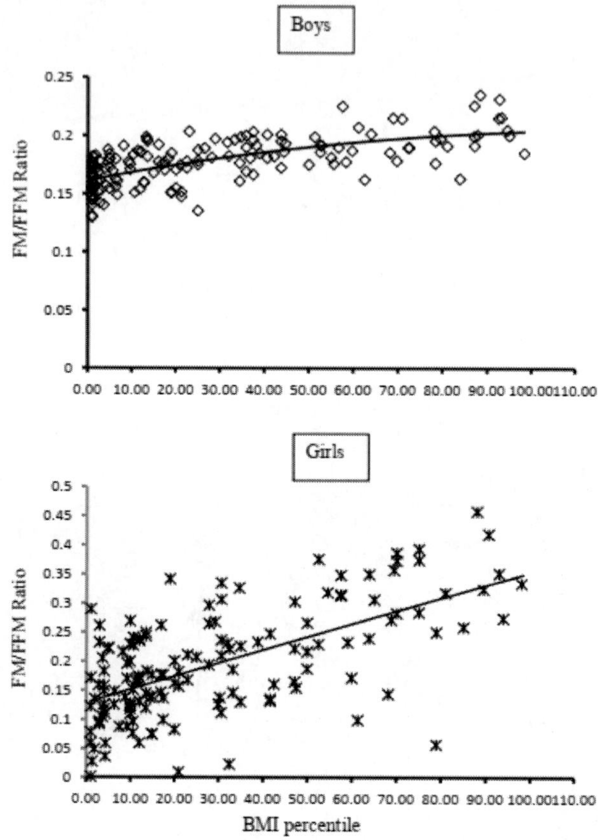

Figure 8. Individual data points of fat mass (FM)/fat free mass (FFM) ratio against BMI percentile for age (a) and (b) for boys and girls respectively.

TRACKING OF THIN-FAT PHENOTYPE

The weight for height indices such as Z-scores have not been evaluated for their ability to predict FFM. Weight for height and recently introduced body mass index (BMI) Z-score for children do not distinguish fat and fat free masses. In fact there is a twofold range of variation in fatness for a given BMI value in individual children (Wells & Fewtrell, 2006). Based on skin fold measurement Yajnik and Colleagues have shown that Indian babies are not only small but also have less muscle mass and relatively more fat mass,

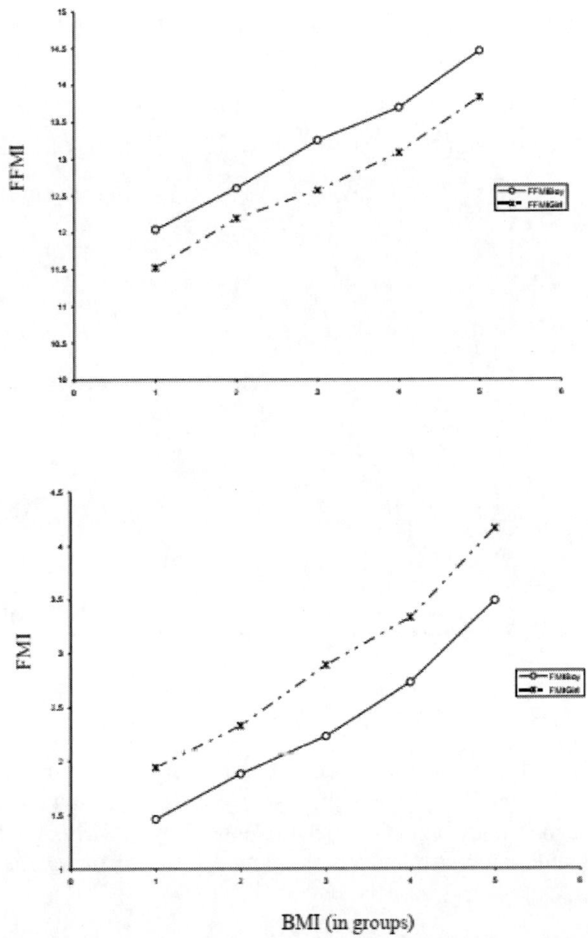

Figure 9. Mean data points for FFMI and FMI derived by the new equation of the study children (n=328) are plotted against BMI in groups (BMI 12 to <14=1, BMI 14 to <15=2, BMI 15 to <16=3, BMI 16 to <17 =4 & BMI ≥ 17=5). —✳— represents girls and --ө--- represents boys.

the so called 'thin fat baby' syndrome (Yajnik et al., 2002, 2003). They further showed that thin fat babies grow up to become thin fat adults with thinner limbs and high waist-hip ratio; they appear to be foetally programed and predisposed to diabetes. He also showed that the smallness and thinness of Indian babies is present at birth and an unusual thin-fat baby composition is associated with the insulin resistance syndrome (Yajnik et al., 2002,

2003). To further understand and study such phenomena validated prediction equations for FFM based on anthropometry should be of value. The conventional weight for height indices and BMI percentile are likely to be inadequate to understand the growth and development of FFM.

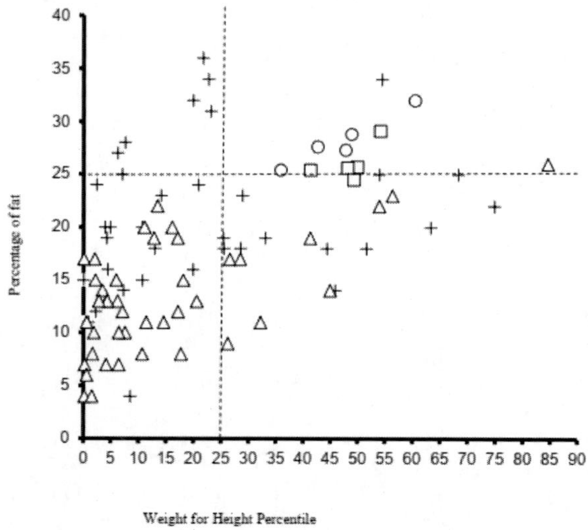

Figure 10. Individual data points for percentage of body fat (% body fat) derived by D_2O dilution reference method (Boys Δ, girls +) are plotted against weight for height percentile. The mean % body fat of American infants (Boys □, girls o) of the same age group derived by multicomponent models are plotted against their weight for height percentiles.

Babies in South Asia have a lower birth weight than their western counterparts, and studies have shown that body-fat is relatively preserved in these babies leading to their description as 'thin fat' (Yajnik et al., 2003). Further adult populations in India have a higher percentage of body fat for a given BMI than Western populations (Krishnaveni et al., 2005, Bavedkar, 1999). Based on the above, it has been speculated that increased body fat at birth tracks into adulthood depending on environmental constraints (Muthayya et al., 2006). This study has generated quality data on fat and lean body mass percentage in a group of infants from low-middle income families. On examining the association of the percentage of fat in our study infants (Figure 10) with leanness as indicated by their weight-for-length percentile, we note that 55 (17%) of the 331 children are below 25th percentile for weight for length by the NCHS standard who may be consider lean. Of these 55 infants, 6(11%) had more than 25% body fat. Therefore, nearly 11% of the lean infants had high fat percentage who may be considered to fall among the so called thin-fat phenotype as described by Yajnik and Collegues (Yajnik et al., 2003).

CONCLUSION

We used a stable isotope dilution technique as the reference standard. Isotope dilution methods use a two component model to measure FFM and FM and are generally safe, reliable, accurate and feasible in infants and children.

The BIA is a simple and suitable method as an epidemiological tool and is the only practical method that estimates FFM.

The validated published equations and the new equations should go a long way in fulfilling the need for in-depth studies to understand the early origin (i.e., fetal, neonatal and early childhood) of adult diseases of great public health importance such as, diabetes, hypertension, coronary heart disease.

Based on skin-fold measurement, Yajnik and Colleagues, 2003 have shown that Indian babies are not only small at birth they also have less muscle mass and relatively more fat mass, the so called 'thin fat baby' syndrome (Yajnik et al, 2002; 2003). They further showed that thin fat babies grow up to become thin fat adults with thinner limbs and high waist-hip ratio; they appear to be foetally programed and predisposed to diabetes. He also showed that the smallness and thinness of Indian babies is present at birth and an unusual thin-fat body composition is associated with the insulin resistance syndrome (Yajnik, 2004). To further understand and study such phenomena validated prediction equations for FFM based on BIA should be of great value.

We note that %fat in both boys and girls are generally much lower than those found in healthy American infants of similar age group. However in four girls and one boy the %fat values were higher than the reference data. We examined their weight for age and weight for height standard deviation scores (data not shown) and they were considerably lower than the median reference values (of NCHS reference data for age. Except for these five infants it appears that the study infants do not demonstrates the so-called phenomenon of "thin-fat Indian baby" syndrome described by Yajnik CS and colleagues (Yajnik et al, 2003). It should however be noted that these equations were developed on infants from a relatively low socioeconomic status and they should be applied with caution on infants from high socioeconomic strata in South Asia.

These apparently healthy infants drawn from relatively low socioeconomic strata of a metropolitan city in India are generally very lean. This phenomenon largely reflects inadequate nutrition during infancy and early childhood and is likely to be a consequence of the well known phenomenon of prolonged breast feeding combined with inadequate weaning food of low energy density. The current breastfeeding rate in this study population was as high as 88%.

Until recently, interest in postnatal weight gain was primarily related to causes of failure to thrive, such as malnutrition, infection and other pathological and genetic disorders. However, the situation changed with the recent studies that raised the possibility that rapid postnatal growth may be associated with an increased risk of chronic diseases in adult life such as diabetes, hypertension and coronary heart disease (Baird et al., 2005, Singhal et al., 2004, Metcalf & Monaghan, 2001). In this context the role of breast feeding, particularly prolonged breast feeding as is common in South Asia- should attract a fresh evaluation.

References

Altman DG. (1992). *Practical statistics for medical research.* London: Chapman & Hall. 336-351, 396-402.

Baird J, Fisher D, Lucas P, Kleijnen J, Roberts H, Law C. (2005). Being big or growing fast: systematic review of size and growth in infancy and later obesity. *BMJ*, 331: 929-931.

Barker DJ. (2001). A new model for the origins of chronic disease. *Med Health Care Philos,* 4: 31-35.

Bavedkar A, Yajnik CS, Fall CHD, Bapat S, Pandit AN, Deshpande V et al. (1999). Insulin resistance syndrome in 8-year-old Indian children: small at birth, big at 8 years, or both? *Diabetes,* 48: 2422-2429.

Bocage C. (1988). *Impedance measurement of body composition in children.* MSc. Thesis, University of West Indies, Kingston, Jamaica.

Bulatao RA and Stephens PW. (1992). Global Estimates and projections of Mortality by Cause, 1970-2015. Working paper Series 1007. Washington DC: World Bank.

Butte NF, Hopkinson JM, Wong WW, Smith EO & Ellis KJ. (2000). Body Composition during the First 2 Years of Life: An Updated Reference. *Pediatric Research*, 47(5): 578-585.

Daniels SR. (2006). The consequences of childhood overweight and obesity. *Future child,* 16: 47-67.

Demerath EW, Schubert CM, Maynard LM, Sun SS, Chumlea WC, Pickoff A, Czerwinski SA, Townw B, Siervogel RM. (2006). Do changes in body mass index percentile reflect changes in body composition in children? Data from the Fels Longitudinal study. *Pediatrics,* 117(3): e487-495.

Deurenberg P, van der Kooy K, Leenen R, et al. (1989). Body impedance is largely dependent on the intra- and extra-cellular water distribution. *Eur J ClinNutr,* 43: 845-853.

Deurenberg P, Weststrate JA, Paymans I, et al. (1988). Factors affecting bioelectrical impedance measurements in humans. *Eur J ClinNutr,* 42: 1017-1022.

Eriksson JG, Forsen T, Tuomilehto J, Osmond C and Barker DJ. (2001). Early growth and coronary heart disease in later life: longitudinal study. *BMJ,* 318:427-431.

Eriksson JG, Forsen T, Tuomilehto J, Osmond C, Barker DJ. (2003). Early adiposity rebound in childhood and risk of Type-2 diabetes in adult life. *Diabetologia,* 46: 190-194.

Eriksson JG, Forsen T, Tuomilehto J, Winter PD, Osmond C & Barker DJ. (1999). Catch-up growth in childhood and death from coronary heart disease: longitudinal study. *BMJ,* 318**:** 427-431.

Fall CHD. (2001). Non-industrialised countries and affluence: relationship with type 2 diabetes. *Br.Med Bull,* 60:33-50.

Fjeld CR, Freundt-Thurne J & Schoeller DA. (1990). Total body water measured by ^{18}O dilution and bioelectrical impedance in well and malnourished children. *Pediatr Res,* 27: 98-102.

Frankel S, Elwood P, Sweetnam P, Yarnell J and Davey Smith G. (1996). Birthweight, adult risk factors and incident coronary heart disease: the Caerphilly study. *Public Health,*110:139-43.

Gurav RB, Kartikeyan S, Jape MR. (2003). Low birth weight babies – a pilot study. *BMJ*, 326: 911-915.

Krishnaveni GV, Hill JC, Veena SR, Leary SD, Saperia J, Chachyamma KJ et al. (2005). Truncal adiposity is present at birth and in early childhood in South Indian children. *Indian Pediatr,* 84:527-538.

Kushner RF, Schoeller DA, Fjeld CR, et al. (1992). Is the impedance index (ht^2/R) significant in predicting total body water? *Am J Clin Nutr,* 56: 835-839.

Leibel RL. (2008). Molecular physiology of weight regulation in mice and humans. *Int J Obes* (Lon), 32(suppl 7): S98-S108).

Maynard LM, Wisemandle W, Roche AF, Chumlea WC, Guo SS, Siervogel RM. (2001). Childhood body composition in relation to body mass index. *Pediatrics*, 107:344-350.

Mellits ED & Cheek DB. (1970). The assessment of body water and fatness from infancy to adulthood. *Monograph of the Society for Research in Child development,* 35(7): 12-26.

Metcalfe NB, Monaghan P. (2001). Compensation for a bad start: grow now, pay later*? Trends Ecol Evol*, 16(5): 254-260.

Morgenstern BZ, Mahoney DW & Warady BA. (2002). Estimating Total Body Water in children on the basis of Height and Weight: A

Reevaluation of the Formulas of Mellits & Cheek. *J Am Soc Nephrol*, 13(7): 1884-1888.

Muthayya S. (2009). Maternal nutrition & low birth weight- what is really important? *Ind. J Med Res,* 130(5):600-608.

Muthyayya S, Dwarknath P, Thomas T, Vaz M, Mhaskar A, Mhaskar R et al. (2006). Anthropometry and body composition of South Indian babies at birth. *Public Health Nutr,* 9(7): 896-903.

Nyboer J. (1972). Workable volume and flow concepts of bio-segments by electrical impedance plethysmography. *TIT J Life Sci,* 21-13.

Osmond C, Barker DJ, Winter PD, Fall CHD and Simmonds SJ. (1993). Early growth and death from cardiovascular disease in women. *BMJ,* 307(6918):1519-1524.

Rich-Edward JW, Stampfer MJ, Manson JE, Rosner B, Hankinson SE, Colditz GA, Willetl WC, Hennekens CH. (1997). Birth weight and risk of cardiovascular disease in a cohort of women followed up since 1976. *BMJ,* 315:396-400.

Rolland-Cachera MF, Deheeger M, Guilloud-Bataille M, Avons P, Patois E, Sempe M. (1987). Tracking the development of adiposity from one month of age to adulthood. *Ann Hum Bio*, 14(3):219-229.

Sen A, Mahalanabis D, Mukhopadhyay S, Chakrabarty K, Singh AK, Bisai S, Chakarbarty M, Halder D, Islam MA. (2005). Routine use of antimicrobials by pregnant Indian women does not improve birth outcome: a randomized controlled trial. *J Health Popul Nutr*, 23(3): 236-244.

Sen B, Mahalanabis D, Kurpad AV, Shaikh S, Bose K. (2010). Total body water and fat free mass: evaluation of equations based on bioelectrical impedance analysis in infants and young children in India. *Br J Nutr,* 104(2): 256-264.

Sen B, Mahalanabis D, Shaikh S, et al. (2009). Evaluation of equations for fat free mass based on anthropometry in infants and young children in South Asia. *Br J Nutr,* 101(4): 551-557.

Sen B, Mahalanabis D. (2017). Development of prediction equations for body composition in Indian children using bioelectrical impedance analysis. *Coll. Antropol*, 4: 253-260.

Singhal A, Cole TJ, Fewtrell M, Deanfield J, Lucas A. (2004). Is slower early growth beneficial for long-term cardiovascular health? *Circulation,* 109: 1108-1113.

Unicef. (2012). The state of the world's children. *Children in an urban world,* 92-93.

Van Itallie TB, Yang MU, Heymsfield SB, Funk RC, Boileau R. (1990). Height- normalized indices of the body's fat-free mass and fat mass: potentially useful indicators of nutritional status. *Am J Clin Nutr* 52: 953-459.

Wells JCK &Fewtrell MS. (2006). Measuring body composition. *Arch Dis Child,* 91: 612-617.

Wild S, Roglic G, Green A, Sicree R and King H. (2004). Global prevalence of diabetes: estimate for the year 2000 and projections for 2030. *Diabetes Care,* 27: 1047-1053.

Yajnik CS, Fall CH, Coyaji KJ et al. (2003). Neonatal anthropometry: The thin-fat Indian baby. The Pune Maternal Nutrition Study. *International Journal of Obesity and Related Metabolic Disorders*, 27(2):173-180.

Yajnik CS, Lubree HG, Rege SS et al. (2002). Adiposity and Hyper-insulinemia in Indians are present at birth. *Journal of Clinical Endocrinol & Metab,* 87: 5575-5580.

In: Contemporary Issues in Childhood … ISBN: 978-1-53617-348-2
Editors: J. Ratan Ghosh and K. Bose ©2020 Nova Science Publishers, Inc.

Chapter 6

Environmental and Genetic Factors Affecting Body Mass and Proportion among Individuals on the Progressive Stages of Ontogenesis in Poland (Central Europe)

Paulina Pruszkowska-Przybylska*
Department of Anthropology,
Faculty of Biology and Environmental Protection,
University of Łódź, Poland

Abstract

Body mass and proportions disorders are now a global problem on every stage of the human ontogenesis, not only among adults but also among children. Causes of these disorders are extensive and ambiguous. However, the main groups of factors connected with body mass and proportions disorders are the following: genetic and environmental factors

* Corresponding Author's Email: paulina.pruszkowska@biol.uni.lodz.pl.

including lifestyle, prenatal period, and socio-economical status. Epigenetics provides new information, which links genetic and environmental influences. Consequence of it are chemical modifications of DNA without changing quantity and order of nucleotides.

INTRODUCTION

Body composition and proportion disorders among children are nowadays very important issues. Regarding the rising problem of obesity but also underweight more studies are needed in this area. The mentioned problems are important for human population on every stage of ontogenesis. In both cases - obesity and underweight, the influence of various socioeconomic, genetic and environmental factors is observed. To appropriately recognise type of the body composition and proportion disorders it is crucial to distinguish their direct and indirect genesis. These body composition and proportion disorders which directly result from conscious manipulation of the daily energy balance and those which indirectly result from other diseases. This type of categorization has particular importance in clinical practice, diagnosis and therapy (Table 1).

Table 1. Division of deficiencies and excess body mass with respect to causes (Myszkowska-Ryciak et al., 2012; Kuczmarski et al., 2000; Lewitt et al., 2008; Męczekalski et al., 2008).

Direct (primary)		**Indirect (secondary)**	
Deficiencies	Excess	Deficiencies	Excess
• Anorexia nervosa • Bulimia nervosa	• Overweight • Obesity	• Advanced stage of AIDS • Tuberculosis • Cancer	• Syndromes: -Prader -Willi, -Bardet -Biedl, -Alstrom and Cohe

UNDERWEIGHT (DEFINITION, TYPES, CAUSES)

Body mass deficiencies may have a different genesis, most often they are an effect (conscious or unconscious) of supplying insufficient amount of energy values in relation to energy expenditure for a given individual (appropriate for age, sex, type of physical activity). The conscious achievement of a body mass deficit is understood as manipulation of the energy balance, obtained through the use of reducing diets and physical exercises. The unconscious attainment of a lack of body mass results from limited material resources, the lack of sufficient resources to provide the individual with an adequate amount of a full-fledged diet.

The group of body weight deficits achieved consciously includes anorexia nervosa (AN) and bulimia nervosa (BN). The AN is a psychical disorder which is characterized by restrictive abandonment of the amount of food consumed. In contrast to AN patients suffering from BN do not reduce food consumption, but after meal they remove food introduced into the digestive system in a direct way by using vomiting or laxatives, or indirectly through forceful physical exercises (Strzelecki et al., 2007).

Statistical Data Showing the Problem of Underweight at Selected Stages of Ontogenesis

According to Hoeke (2006) 8 out of every 100,000 people suffer AN in one year. In the years 1935-1999 an upward trend in the number of people diagnosed with AN is observed, most often these are women aged 15 to 24 years. The average incidence of AN among girls and young women is 0.3%, while BN is 1%.

The problem of children and young people with underweight is worth to explain giving as an example country from central Europe - Poland.

Based on the available sources it is known that the percentage of people with body weight deficits varies depending on the region of Poland and depending on the calendar age of the subjects (ontogenesis stage). In Eastern Poland, 14.9% of girls aged 10-15 years belong to the group of children with weight deficiencies (Popławska et al., 2011). In Northern Poland, deficiencies in body mass (Walentukiewicz et al., 2011) are observed in 14% of girls aged 18 years. Less often, body mass deficiencies are observed in children living in the Western regions of the country - in the group of 10-15 year-old boys, the prevalence is 9.6%, among girls - 11.5% (Czajka and Kochan, 2012). Among the students of Central Poland, weight loss is observed in 11% of people (Kardjalik et al., 2012).

According to research by Żądzińska et al., (2012), conducted in 2002/2004 among children and young people living in Lodz, the problem of underweight concerns 13.7% of boys in the 7-12 age group, 12.5% in the 13-15 age group and 8.7% in group of 16-18 years. In the group of girls, underweight is observed much more frequently. Among 7-12 year olds, body weight deficits were found in 23.6% of girls, in girls 13-15 years - 20.2% and 17.7% in girls aged 16-18. These results were compared with data obtained in studies conducted in Lodz in the years 1977/1978, 1987/1988, 1992/1994. In the years 1977/1978 the prevalence of underweight in both sexes was higher than a decade later. Since 1987, there has been a clear trend of increasing frequency of body weight deficits in children of both sexes, in all age categories.

Definitely less unified data on the above topic applies to older age groups. According to the studies by Szklarska and Lipowicz (2012) this specific "gap" in research may be partly caused by the awareness of the consequences of measurement error resulting from the fact that body weight decreases with age as a result of lowering bone mineral density (additionally it is a feature that is influenced by age, sex and lifestyle, i.e., smoking, drinking coffee, alcohol consumption, physical activity, education level, as well as the number of born children in the case of women).

How Genes Affect Underweight?

The development of molecular biology has significantly influenced the search for causes of body mass deficiencies that are the consequence of AN and BN in the human genome. The most frequently mentioned genes connected with AN and BN are: CNR1 encoding endocannabinoid CB1 receptor, FAAH gene coding fatty acid amide hydrolase (Monteleone et al., 2009) and 5-HTT gene - serotonin transporter (Castellini et al., 2012).

The polymorphism rs1049353 (G / A) of the CNR1 gene shows an increased incidence in patients with AN and BM. In patients with AN, the synergistic effect of the gene polymorphisms CNR1 - rs1049353 (G/A) and FAAH rs324420 (C/A) was more frequent, while no such effect was observed in patients with BM.

Among patients with AN and BN, disturbed serotonin activity is observed which, according to research, may be responsible for modulation of abnormal nutritional behaviors. The gene encoding the serotonin transporter is an integral membrane protein located in the presynaptic neuronal membrane. The 5-HTT protein is encoded by a single gene located on the 17th chromosome (Calati et al., 2011).

There are described 50 polymorphisms at the 5-HTT gene promoter sites (Castellini et al., 2012). One of these 5-HTTLPR is located in the transcriptional control region at the 5 'end of the 5-HTTLPR coding sequence. It is composed of 43 base pairs (bp) of repeating 6 or 8 elements undergoing insertion or deletion. The case with deletions is the short version (S), while the insertions decide on the long variant (L). The occurrence of the S variant reduces the transcriptional performance of the 5-HTT gene promoter, which in turn increases the expression of the 5-HTT gene. A higher frequency of the S variant is observed in patients with AN compared to healthy subjects, however, this relationship was not found among patients with BN (Calati et al., 2011). As the researches show in the group of patients with AN excessive activity of some areas of the brain responsible for the production of serotonin was also noticed (Bailer et al., 2005).

The significance of genetic factors in the epidemiology of the formation of consciously controlled body mass deficits is supported by research indicating the more frequently observed diseases of eating disorders associated with body mass deficiencies in both monozygotic twins (Suisman et al., 2012).

Association of Environmental Factors with Underweight

Reports about environmental factors that have a significant impact on the prevalence of body weight deficiencies are numerous, including place of residence, level of education, impact of previous illnesses (Larsen et al., 2018). The environment is understood as a set of external factors affecting the genotype by shaping the phenotype of the organism. Among the most frequently analyzed environmental factors which significantly modify the body mass, are: lifestyle, socio-economic status, level of environmental pollution and also the prenatal environment.

Mass culture is a significant factor shaping the attitudes of the society, including the choice of a lifestyle that may maintain the development of eating disorders that lead to body mass deficiencies, especially in the group of young girls (Strzelecki et al., 2007).

In order to achieve the intended goal some girls follow the cultural trends changing their lifestyle. In some cases the consequence of this may be BN (gluttony attacks intertwined with periods of hunger, patients after the meal make use of vomiting, diuretic measures, as well as increased physical exercise) or AN (patients use restrictive diets and intense physical activity). Researches indicate that eating disorders mainly affect females (Frąckowiak-Sochańska, 2011, Strzelecki et al., 2007).

There is little information about the correlation of prenatal environment conditions with the tendency to suffer from diseases resulting in low body mass in postnatal life. However, according to Mathieu (2009) women suffering from pregorexia through the use of food restrictions may affect the child's body mass defects as well as underweight. Moreover in the research conducted by Żądzińska and Rosset (2013) they proved that children whose mothers experienced trauma during pregnancy were more frequent underweight in comparison with children whose mothers were not affected by trauma during pregnancy.

As the research shows, there is a statistically significant relationship between socioeconomic status and the probability of developing an AN. A higher socioeconomic status predisposes to the disease (Ziora et al., 2008, Lewitt et al., 2008) what was proposed on the basis of the research conducted on the selected group of Polish patients (Ziora et al., 2008). The factors that testified to the higher socio-economic status in the studies were the residential conditions of the patients. The largest number of patients declared single-family houses or new apartments as a place of residence. The family model most often found in patients (but also in healthy ones) consists of four members: mother, father and two children. In the families of patients the presence of grandparents living in the family home was also frequently found, which according to Ziora et al., (2008) may indicate a single-family house as a place of residence, because multi-generational families usually live in a single-family homes. Among the patients, more frequent occurrence of family-related conflicts was observed, as well as the origin of patients from single-parent families (Ziora et al., 2008, Lewitt et al., 2008).

OVERWEIGHT AND OBESITY (DEFINITION, TYPES, CAUSES)

In terms of excess weight, overweight and obesity of I, II and III type are distinguished. Overweight and obesity are the main clinical problems of modern human populations resulting from eating disorders. The distinction between these two diseases is made on the basis of the individual BMI index related to the range of variation of this trait that is appropriate for the age and sex of the subject (Kuczmarski et al., 2000; Rosset et al., 2009). Obesity is defined by WHO (WHO, 2000) as abnormal and extensive accumulation of fat that negatively affects human health.

Due to the different type of adipose tissue localization we distinguish: femoral-gluteal obesity (more often diagnosed in women), and abdominal, visceral obesity (more frequent in men as well as in postmenopausal women) (Staroń et al., 2005).

Statistical Data Showing the Problem of Overweight and Obesity at Selected Stages of Ontogenesis

Due to the significant increase in the frequency of people with excess body mass in each age group, in all human populations in 2004 WHO declared a world-wide epidemic of obesity (Sikorska-Wiśniewska 2007). Since then, more and more research has been conducted into the causes of this phenomenon (Żądzinska et al., 2004, Janssen et al., 2005, Sikorska-Wiśniewska, 2007, Sitek et al., 2012). According to Eriksson et al., (2003), the risk factors of obesity include the birth weight and body mass achieved in the first years of life and during the child's puberty - 80% of obese children in childhood have a lifetime of problems (Osiecka-Chojnacka, 2012).

In Europe, 10-25% of men and 10-30% of women struggle with excess body mass. Over the past 10 years, the prevalence of obesity has increased by 10-40% depending on the population. Over 50% of the European society are people with excess body mass. In addition, higher-than-expected BMI is more common in men than in women (Tsigos et al., 2009). According to a cross-sectional study of young people (10-16 years) from 34 (mainly European) participating countries in the 2001-2002 Health Behavior in School-Aged Study, the highest incidence of excess body weight (overweight and obesity) has been observed in Malta (25, 4% and 7.9%) and in the United States (25.1% and 6.8%). The lowest frequency of excess body weight was found in Lithuania (5.1% and 0.4%) and Latvia (5.9% and 0.5%). The prevalence of overweight and obesity is particularly high in North America, southwestern Europe and the United Kingdom (Janssen et al., 2005). According to data from 2008, Malta was overtaken by the British Isles in terms of the frequency of excess body mass (Osiecka-Chojnacka, 2012).

In Poland, based on various studies, differences in the frequency of diagnosed excess weight of children might be observed also on regional level. In Eastern Poland, 8.6% of girls in pubertal age (here, examined girls aged 10-15 years) belong to the group with excess body weight, overweight is characterized by 7.9% of girls, and 0.7% by obesity (Popławska et al.,

2011). In Northern Poland, 16% of girls aged 18 show excessive body mass (Walentukiewicz et al., 2011). In the group of boys aged 10-15 living in Western Poland, 16.8% are overweight children and 5% are obese. In the group of girls from this region of the country, 13.1% of children are overweight, 4.3% are obese (Czajka, Kochan 2012). Among students of Central Poland, 26.6% of men and 6.5% of women (Kardjalik et al., 2012) belong to the group of people with excess body mass. According to the aforementioned studies, Żądzińska et al., (2012), conducted in 2002/2004 among children and adolescents living in Lodz, overweight concerns 17.4% of boys in the 7-12 age group, 17.0% in the 13-15 age group and 15.9% in 16-18 age group. However, in the group of Lodz's girls, 13.5% of children aged 7-12, 12.6% aged 13-15 and 8.1% aged 16-18 are characterized by excess body weight. The above values compared with the results obtained in studies from the previous three decades (from 1977/1978, 1987/1988, 1992/1994) show that in all 4 studies conducted, the percentage of girls with overweight is similar, the exception is increased 7-12 year old girls with overweight in 1992/1994. In the group of boys, the picture is slightly different. Most cases of overweight concerned boys 7-12 years old in 1977/1978, while in 1987/1988 a decrease to 14.5% was recorded, and in 1992/1994 and 2002/2004 a further increase to 17.4% for this group age. In the age range of 13-15 years, in the years 1977/1978, 1987/1988, 1992/1994, a downward trend was observed (1977/1978 - 16.4%, 1987/1988 - 15.9%, 1992 / 1994 - 13.2%) in the 2002/2004 study, the number of overweight boys increased again (17.0%) in the oldest group (16-18 years). The smallest problem of overweight was registered in 1987/1988 (8.4%), in 1977/1978 (12.0%) it was higher than in 1987/1988, but smaller than in 1992/1994 and 2002/2004 when the upward trend was observed (respectively 15.3% and 15.9%).

How Genes Affect Overweight and Obesity?

Obesity is a trait determined by many genes, only 200 cases of monogenic obesity have been described globally (Męczekalski, 2008). Current research based on twins revealed that genetic predisposition explained the 47% to 80% BMI variation (Elks et al., 2012). Silventoinen et al., (2010) demonstrated that the BMI of adopted children correlates strongly with biological parents, and less with adoptive parents. The gene most frequently mentioned in the literature which include the highest number of polymorphisms predisposing to fat accumulation is FTO. The FTO gene is located on the long arm of the 16 chromosome (16q12.2) and encodes the enzyme - 2-oxoglutarate demethylase, occurring e.g., in the hypothalamus. It is responsible for the craving and spending of energy, probably by affecting the intensity of lipolysis in adipocytes, it can induce the amount of adipose tissue (Sitek et al., 2014). The polymorphism rs9939609 of this gene is an important predisposing factor to obesity (Wåhlén et al., 2008).

Researchers are wondering why humans evolved genes determining predisposition to obesity. It is possible that this is a legacy of ancestors who, due to their nomadic lifestyle, did not have constant access to food. Therefore, individuals that were able to accumulate the largest resources of food consumed were evolutionarily better adapted to the environment, and thus to survive and transfer "sparing" genes to descendants (Kapka-Skrzypczak, 2012). A change in lifestyle has caused a growing problem of a balanced energy balance. Food became more easily available so energy costs related to obtaining food were minimized. In addition, in modern human populations a decrease in physical activity is observed in favor of passive rest (Osiecka-Chojnacka, 2012).

Association of Environmental Factors and Increased Body Mass

The formation of processes that result in excess body mass depends on the complex interactions between genetic determinant, diet, physical activity and the living environment as a factor composed of many interdependent elements - variables (physical, social-economic, cultural), whose outcome may condition the above disorders (Papas et al., 2007).

Lifestyle

Physical activity seems to be the most important environmental factor modifying excess body weight (Kozieł et al., 2006; Papas et al., 2007). The most disturbing are studies indicating the lack of physical activity among children and adolescents. According to data collected as part of the project "2001-2002 Health Behavior in School-Aged Study" (Janssen et al., 2005) in most countries of the world with children diagnosed overweight or obesity, the level of physical activity was lower and the time of watching TV longer compared to children with normal body mass. In addition, in 91% of the countries surveyed the higher frequency of consumption of sweets was associated with excess weight.

According to studies by Kulińska-Szukalska and Chlebny-Sokół (2011) on a group of 102 children aged 10-15 years residing in Poland their physical activity is very small, the majority of children prefer a sedentary lifestyle. Their diet is often incorrectly balanced, contains too much fat (including cholesterol) and carbohydrates, and too little proteins. Parents' eating habits seem to be significant. Children growing up among obese family members (who are probably characterized by bad eating habits) are more prone to overweight or obesity. Over the years, quantitative and qualitative changes in the amount of food consumed are noted, it is high-energy food with negligible nutritional value, highly processed eaten at irregular times of the day (Osiecka-Chojnacka, 2012).

Thanks to Vaaga et al., (2012) it is known that an important factor that may affect the development of post-natal obesity is the poorly balanced diet of the mother in the prenatal period of the child. When the mother does not provide the right amount of nutrients the developing fetus "remembers" the fact of rare food intake and tries to accumulate as much energy stocks as possible. In addition, it probably leads to epigenetic changes and in the postnatal period the body operates in the same way, according to the rule of economical phenotype, leading to obesity, as well as to grade II diabetes or metabolic syndrome (Hales and Barker 2001, Cameron and Demerath 2002, Wells, 2007, 2012). Moreover sex hormones in prenatal period can be also connected with body composition in the future life. The 2D:4D digit ratio is known as an indicator of fat and muscle mass due to the fact that it is as a result of prenatal exposure to sex hormones along with the rule that the higher index value the higher concentration of prenatal female sex hormones and the lower index value the higher concentration of prenatal male sex hormones. Additionally, it is widely known that testosterone affects muscle mass growth and that oestrogen maintains adipogenesis. Pruszkowska-Przybylska et. al. (2018) proved that the digit ratio is negatively associated with muscle mass among girls what may be an important information in creating the obesity prevention programs.

Socio-Economic Status

Global trends indicate a higher rate of obesity in well developed countries with lower socio-economic status, but within these populations a higher SES (socio-economic status) seems to be a protective factor against excess body weight (Manios et al., 2018). Probably knowledge and awareness about healthy lifestyle of families characterized by higher socio-economic status (in this group parents have higher education) affects the described effect (Osiecka-Chojnacka, 2012). In turn, in families with a lower SES especially with parental elementary education, the lack of funds for the purchase of healthy food and active spending of free time causes the observed increase in the frequency of children with excess weight (Kozieł et al., 2001). The researches show that the greater the diversification of the socio-economic status, the larger the group of people with excess body mass in the studied population (Osiecka-Chojnacka, 2012).

Noteworthy in Central and Eastern Europe, the period of political transformation (the turn of the 1980s and 1990s) was reversed (high SES correlated with childhood overweight and obesity) (Kozieł et al., 2000; Kozieł et al., 2004; Żądzińska et al., 2012; Gomuła et al., 2015). Ulijaszek and Koziel (2007) explain these phenomena decreasing of physical activity which is connected with higher incomes often spent on such goods as cars, computers, television which are linked with sedentary lifestyle.

EPIGENETICS

For the epidemiology of body proportions, very promising are research results showing that epigenetic changes of the human genome can be connected with body mass. The epigenetics deals with the study of non-genetic heredity, or heredity of gene expression changes independent of the DNA sequence. The mechanisms of epigenetics include: DNA methylation, histone modifications, modifications of non-coding RNA (Jiménez-Chillarón et al., 2012).

According to Jiménez-Chillarón et al., (2012) the type of food consumed has a significant impact on the generation of epigenetic changes. The diets that show the above effects include diets: rich in fats, exceeding daily caloric intake, low in proteins, limiting daily caloric intake, containing polyphenols, biotin, ethanol.

Epigenetic changes may occur at all stages of ontogenesis, however the pre-natal period, especially the period between conception and embryo implantation (the first 8 days of intra-uterine life), seems to be the most eco-positive period. Therefore, the mother's diet is crucial in shaping the morphological and physiological features of the child's body at the subsequent stages of ontogenesis, also determining disturbances in weight-increase proportions, including excess body weight.

The causes of body composition and proportion diseases are the resultant of many environmental and genetic factor. Nonetheless, it is difficult to assess to what extent the genetic variables in which prenatal factors (programming development) correspond to the disturbances of body proportions and in which environmental modifiers (lifestyle, diet, SES). According to the latest research, the value of BMI to a different degree depends on genetic and environmental factors in women and men (Bergin et al., 2012). BMI of women turns out to be more dependent on genetic factors than men (however, environmental factors have a greater impact on the change in BMI). In the case of men, environmental factors seem to be a definite cause of modulation of BMI values. Greater male susceptibility to fluctuation changes in BMI values ay be associated with greater ecosensitivity, characteristic of this sex (Janiszewska et al., 2012).

Table 2. Characteristics of epigenetic modifications (Jiménez-Chillarón et al., 2012, Mehler, 2008)

DNA methylation	**Modifications of histones**	**Modifications of non-coding RNA (ncRNA, non-coding RNA)**
This is a covalent modification based on the addition of methyl groups to cosine. It occurs above all on CpG dinucleotides. CpG islands are regions in DNA that have a very large number of Cp G dinucleotides (mainly areas near the promoter).	These are series of complex post-translational modifications: • mono-, di-trimerylations • phosphorylation, • glycosylation, • ubiquitination • ADP-ribosylation	It involves increased transcriptional activity from two DNA strands, non-coding regions. The obtained transcripts determine the presence of non-coding regulatory RNAs.

REFERENCES

Bailer U. F., Guido K. F., Shannan E. H., Price J. C., Meltzer C. C, Weissfeld L., Mathis C. H., Drevets W. C, Wagner A., Hoge J., Ziolko S. K., McConaha C. W., Kaye W. H. 2005. Brain Serotonin 5-HT1A Receptor Binding after recovery from anorexia nervosa measured by positron emission tomographyand [Carbonyl11C] WAY-100635. *Archives of General Psychiatry*, 62 (9): 1032-1041.

Bergin J. E., Neale M. C., Eaves L. J., Martin N. G., Heath A. C., Maes H. H. 2012. Genetic and Environmental Transmission of Body Mass Index Fluctuation. *Behavior Genetics*, 42(6): 867-874.

Calati R., Ronchi D., Bellini M., Serretti A. 2011. The 5-HTTLPR polymorphism and eating disorders: A meta-analysis. *International Journal of Eating Disorders*, 44 (3): 191–199.

Cameron N., Demerath E. W. 2002. Critical periods in human growth and their relationship to diseases of ageing. *Yearbook Phys. Anthropol.* 45: 159-184

Castellini G., Ricca V., Lelli L., Bagnoli S., Faravelli E. L. C., Sorbi S., Nacmias B. 2012. Association between serotonin transporter gene polymorphism and eating disorders outcome: A 6-year follow-up study *American Journal of Medical Genetics Part B. Neuropsychiatric Genetics Volume*, 159B (5): 491–500.

Czajka K., Kochan K. 2012. BMI a wybrane zachowania zdrowotne uczniów szkółpodstawowych i gimnazjalnych [BMI and selected health behaviors of students of primary and junior high schools] *Problemy Higieny i Epidemiologii [Problems of Hygiene and Epidemiology]*, 93 (3): 551-557.

Elks, C. E., Den Hoed, M., Zhao, J. H., Sharp, S. J., Wareham, N. J., Loos, R. J., & Ong, K. K. (2012). Variability in the heritability of body mass index: a systematic review and meta-regression. *Frontiers in endocrinology*, 3, 29.

Eriksson J., Forse T., Osmond C., Barker D., 2003 Obesity from cradle to grave International. *Journal of Obesity*, 27: 722–727.

Frąckowiak- Sochańska M. 2011. Zdrowie psychiczne kobiet i mężczyzn. Płeć społeczno-kulturowa a kategorie "zdrowia psychicznego" i "chorób psychicznych." [Mental health of men and women. Socio-cultural gender and the categories of "mental health" and "mental illness."] *Nowiny Lekarskie [Medical News]*, 80 (5): 394–406.

Gomula, A., Nowak-Szczepanska, N., Danel, D. P., & Koziel, S. 2015. Overweight trends among Polish schoolchildren before and after the transition from communism to capitalism. *Economics & Human Biology*, 19: 246-257.

Hales C. N., Barker D. J. P. 2001. The thrifty phenotype hypothesis. *Br. Med. Bull.* 60: 5-20.

Hoek HW. 2006. Incidence, prevalence and mortality of anorexia nervosa and other eating disorders. *Current Opinion in Psychiatry*, 19 (4): 389-394.

Janiszewska R. 2012. Wskaźniki rozwoju fizycznego noworodków radomskich urodzonych w różnym wieku płodowym [Indicators of physical development of Radom newborns born at different fetal age]. *Problemy Higieny i Epidemiologii* [Problems of Hygiene and Epidemiology], 93 (4): 702-706.

Janssen P., Katzmarzyk T., Boyce W. F., Vereecken C., Mulvihill C., Roberts C., Currie C., Pickett W. 2005. The Health Behaviour in School-Aged Children Obesity Working Group. Comparison of overweight and obesity prevalence in school-aged youth from 34 countries and their relationships with physical activity and dietary patterns. *Obesity Reviews*, 6 (2): 123–132.

Jiménez-Chillarón J. C., Díaz R., Martínez D., Pentinat T., Ramón-Krauel M., Ribó S., Plösch T. 2012. The role of nutrition on epigenetic modifications and their implications on health. *Biochimie*, 94: 2242-2263.

Kapka-Skrzypczak L., Biliński P., Niedźwiecka J., Kulpa P., Skowron J., Wojtyła A. 2012. Zmiana stylu życia człowieka jako metoda prewencji przewlekłych chorób niezakaźnych [Change of human lifestyle as a method of prevention of chronic non-communicable diseases]. *Problemy Higieny i Epidemiologii* [*Problems of Hygiene and Epidemiology*], 93 (1): 27-31.

Kardjalik K., Bryła M., Maniecka-Bryła I. 2012. Zachowania zdrowotne związane z odżywianiem orazwystępowanie nadwagi i otyłości w grupie studentów [Nutritional health behaviors and the occurrence of overweight and obesity in a group of students]. *Problemy Higieny i Epidemiologii* [*Problems of Hygiene and Epidemiology*], 93 (1): 71-79.

Kuklińska-Szukalska, K., Chlebna-Sokół, D. 2011. Styl życia a występowanie otyłości w badanej grupie dzieci łódzkich [Lifestyle and occurrence of obesity in the studied group of children from Łódź], *Przegląd pediatryczny* [*Pediatric Review*], 41 (4): 152-158.

Kuczmarski R. J., Flegal K. M. 2000. Criteria for definition of overweight in transition: background andrecommendations for the United States. *Special Article The American Journal of Clinical Nutrition*, 72: 1074–1081.

Kozieł, S., Kołodziej, H., & Ulijaszek, S. J. 2000. Parental education, body mass index and prevalence of obesity among 14-year-old boys between 1987 and 1997 in Wrocław, Poland. *European journal of epidemiology*, 16(12): 1163-1167.

Kozieł, S., Welon, Z., Bielicki, T., Szklarska, A., & Ulijaszek, S. 2004. The effect of the economic transition on the body mass index of conscripts in Poland. *Economics & Human Biology*, 2(1): 97-106.

Kozieł, S., Szklarska, A., Bielicki, T., & Malina, R. M. 2006. Changes in the BMI of Polish conscripts between 1965 and 2001: secular and socio-occupational variation. *International journal of obesity*, 30(9): 1382-1388.

Larson, N., Chen, Y., Wall, M., Winkler, M. R., Goldschmit, A. B., & Neumark-Sztainer, D. (2018). Personal, behavioral, and environmental predictors of healthy weight maintenance during the transition to adulthood. *Preventive medicine*, 113, 80-90.

Lewitt A., Brzęczek K., Krupienicz A. 2006. Interwencje żywieniowe w leczeniu anoreksji – wskazówki dietetyczne. *Endokrynologia, Otyłość i Zaburzenia Przemiany Materii*, 4 (3): 128–136.

Manios, Y., Androutsos, O., Katsarou, C., Vampouli, E. A., Kulaga, Z., Gurzkowska, B., Moreno, L. A. (2018). Prevalence and sociodemographic correlates of overweight and obesity in a large Pan-European cohort of preschool children and their families. The ToyBox-study. *Nutrition*.

Mathieu J. 2009. *Topic of professional interest: What Is Pregorexia?*, 109: 974-977.

Mehler M. F. 2008. Epigenetic Principles and Mechanisms Underlying Nervous. System Functions in Health and Disease. *Prog Neurobiol.* 86(4): 305–341.

Męczekalski B., Czyżyk A., Warenik-Szymankiewicz A. 2008. Rola genów w powstawaniu otyłości. Współczesne poglądy, patogeneza, aspekty kliniczne [The role of genes in the formation of obesity. Contemporary views, pathogenesis, clinical aspects]. *Endokrynologia, Otyłość i Zaburzenia Przemiany Materii* [*Endocrinology, Obesity and Metabolic Disorders*], 5 (1): 27–37.

Monteleone P., Filippo C. B. M., Gazzerro P., Canestrelli B., Monteleone F., Proto M. C., Di Genio M., Grimaldi C., Maj M. 2009. Brain and Behavior, Association of CNR1 and FAAH endocannabinoid gene polymorphisms with anorexia nervosa and bulimia nervosa: evidence for synergistic effects. *Genes*, 8: 728-732.

Myszkowska-Ryciak J., Leśniak W., Harton A., Gajewska D., Bawa S. 2012. Poziom wiedzy na temat specyficznych zaburzeń odżywiania w wybranych grupach populacyjnych [The level of knowledge about specific eating disorders in selected population groups]. *Bromatologia i Chemia Toksykologiczna* [*Bromatology and Toxicological Chemistry*], XLV (3):827–832.

Osiecka Chojnacka J. 2012. Obesity epidemic. *Infos zagadnienia społeczno-gospodarcze [Infos socio-economic issues]*, 3 (117): 1-4.

Papas M. A., Alberg A. J., Ewing R., Helzlsouer K. J., Gary T. L., Klassen A. C. 2007. The Built Environment and Obesity. *Epidemiol Rev*, 29: 129–143.

Popławska H., Dmitruk A., Hołub W., Wilczewski A. 2011. Niedowaga i nadwaga a sprawność fizyczna dziewcząt ze wschodniej Polski [Underweight and overweight and physical fitness of girls from eastern Poland]. *Zdrowie Publiczne* [*Public health*], 121 (1): 22-26.

Pruszkowska-Przybylska, P., Nieczuja-Dwojacka, J., & Żądzińska, E. (2018). Supplementation of vitamin D after birth affects body size and BMI in Polish children during the first 3.5 years of life-an analysis based on two cohorts measured in the years 1993-1997 and 2004-2008. *Anthropol. Anz.* 74(5): 413–421

Pruszkowska-Przybylska, P., Sitek, A., Rosset, I., Sobalska-Kwapis, M., Słomka, M., Strapagiel, D., & Żądzińska, E. 2018. Association of the 2D: 4D digit ratio with body composition among the Polish children aged 6-13 years. *Early human development*, 124: 26-32.

Rosset I., Roślak M., Grabowska J., Borowska-Strugińska B., Lorkiewicz W., Sitek A., Stolarczyk H., Śmiszkiewicz-Skwarska A., Żądzińska E. 2009. Stan rozwoju fizycznego dzieci i młodzieży miasta Łodzi [w:] Żądzińska E. (red.) 2004. Dziecko Łódzkie. [Normy rozwoju biologicznego. [*The state of physical development of children and youth of the city of Lodz* [*in:*] *Żądzińska E. (ed.) 2004. Baby Lodz. Standards for biological development*] Wyd. UŁ, Łódź.

Silventoinen, K., Rokholm, B., Kaprio, J., & Sørensen, T. I. (2010). The genetic and environmental influences on childhood obesity: a systematic review of twin and adoption studies. *International journal of obesity*, 34(1), 29.

Sikorska-Wiśniewska G. 2007. Nadwaga i otyłość u dzieci i młodzieży, Żywność, Nauka [Overweight and obesity in children and adolescents, Food, Science]. *Technologia Jakość* [*Technology Quality*], 6 (55): 71 – 80.

Sitek, A., Rosset, I., Strapagiel, D., Majewska, M., Ostrowska-Nawarycz, L., & Żądzińska, E. (2014). Association of FTO gene with obesity in Polish schoolchildren. *Anthropologic Al review*, 77(1), 33-44.

Suisman J. L., Shannon M. O'Connor, Sperry S., Thompson J. K., Keel P. K., Burt S. A., Neale M., Boker S., Klump C. S. K. L. 2012. *International Journal of Eating Disorders.* Genetic and environmental influences on thin-ideal internalization, 45 (8): 942–948.

Staroń K., Maruszyński K., Maj J., Basałyga Z. 2005. Otyłość - niezdrowy styl życia człowieka [Obesity - an unhealthy lifestyle]. *Annales Universitatis Mariae Curie- Skłodowska Lublin-Polonia*, LX(XVI): 244-248.

Strzelecki W., Cybulski M., Strzelecka M., Dolczewska-Samela A. 2007. Zmiana wizerunku medialnego kobiety a zaburzenia odżywiania we współczesnym świecie [Changing the media image of a woman and eating disorders in the modern world]. *Nowiny Lekarskie [Medical News*], 76 (2): 173-181.

Szklarska A., Lipowicz A. 2012. BMI, hypertension and low bone mineral density in adult men and women. *HOMO - Journal of Comparative Human Biology*, 63: 282– 291.

Tsigos C., Hainer V., Basdevant A., Finer N., Fried M., Mathus-Vliegen E., Micic D., Maislos M., Roman G., Schutz Y., Toplak H, Zahorska-Markiewicz B. 2009. Postępowanie w otyłości dorosłych: europejskie wytyczne dla praktyki klinicznej. *Endokrynologia, Otyłość i Zaburzenia Przemiany Materii* [Management of adult obesity: European guidelines for clinical practice. Endocrinology, Obesity and Metabolic Disorders], 5 (3): 87-98.

Ulijaszek, S. J., & Koziel, S. 2007. Nutrition transition and dietary energy availability in Eastern Europe after the collapse of communism. *Economics & Human Biology*, 5(3): 359-369.

Vaag A, Grunnet L. G., Arora G. P., Brons C. 2012. The thrifty phenotype hypothesis revisited. *Diabetologia*, 55 (8): 2085-2088.

Wåhlén, K., Sjölin, E., & Hoffstedt, J. (2008). The common rs9939609 gene variant of the fat mass-and obesity-associated gene FTO is related to fat cell lipolysis. *Journal of lipid research*, 49(3), 607-611.

Walentukiewicz A., Łysak. A, Wilk B. 2011. Uwarunkowania zdrowia gdańskich 18-latek – zachowania Zdrowotne [Health determinants of Gdańsk 18-year-old - Keep Health]. *Problemy Higieny i Epidemiologii* [*Problems of Hygiene and Epidemiology*], 92(3): 482-485.

Wells J. C. K. 2007. The thrifty phenotype as an adaptive Materna effect. *Biol. Rev. Camb. Philos. Soc.* 82: 143-172

Wells J. C. K. 2012. Body composition in infants: evidence for developmental programming and techniques for measurement. *Rev. Endocr. Metab. Disord.* 13: 93-101.

World Health Organization. 2000. Obesity: Preventing and Managing the Global Epidemic. *Report of a WHO Consultation*. World Health Organization, Geneva.

Ziora K., Szalecki M., Nogal P., Ustrzycki J., Oświęcimska J., Rojewska K., Pałasz W., Gorczyca P., Lewiński A., Dyduch A. 2008, Uwarunkowania socjoekonomiczne jadłowstrętu psychicznego [Socioeconomic conditions of anorexia nervosa]. *Przegląd Pediatryczny* [*Pediatric Review*], 38 (1): 33-39.

Żądzińska E., Rosset I., Kozieł S., Nawarycz T., Borowska-Struginska B., Lorkiewicza W., Ostrowska-Nawarycz L., Sitek A. 2012. Frequency of under- and overweight among children and adolescents during the economic transition in Poland. *HOMO - Journal of Comparative Human Biology*, 63: 216–232.

Żądzińska, E., & Rosset, I. 2013. Pre-natal and perinatal factors affecting body mass index in pre-pubertal Polish children. *Annals of human biology*, 40(6): 477-484.

In: Contemporary Issues in Childhood … ISBN: 978-1-53617-348-2
Editors: J. Ratan Ghosh and K. Bose ©2020 Nova Science Publishers, Inc.

Chapter 7

Childhood Obesity in Kolkata, India: Trends and Consequences

Susmita Bharati[1], Manoranjan Pal[2], Aditi Bardhan[1], Priyanka Dhara[4] and Premananda Bharati[3,*]

[1]Sociological Research Unit, Indian Statistical Institute, Kolkata, India
[2]Economic Research Unit, Indian Statistical Institute, Kolkata, India
[3]Biological Anthropology Unit, Indian Statistical Institute, Kolkata, India
[4]Department of Anthropology, Visva-Bharati University, Bolpur, Birbhum, WB, India

Abstract

The paper portrays the prevalence of overweight and obesity among (6-10) year children in India and investigates the probable risk factors of childhood obesity. A sample of 5216 children from classes I to IV has been randomly drawn from 20 different public and private schools in Kolkata, India. For further in-depth study, a random subset of 1682 children, has been selected to find out the probable risk factors of childhood obesity.

---

* Corresponding Author's Email: pbharati@gmail.com.

Age and sex specific overweight and obesity are defined as BMI values above 85th and 95th percentiles respectively (WHO, 2006). To see the relationships of obesity with different factors, chi-square tests, ANOVA and categorical logistic regression have been carried out.

The study reveals that the prevalence of overweight or obese children are 32.4 percent. The children of private schools are more obese than public schools. Different factors like durations of television watching, indoor and out-door games, consumption of junk food items, inheritance pattern and morbidity are the risk factors for childhood obesity.

INTRODUCTION

Obesity is one of the major determinants of morbidity and mortality in many areas of the world. It causes diseases like type 2 diabetes, hypertension and cardiovascular diseases. According to World Health Organization (WHO, 2000), obesity is the cluster of non communicable diseases called "new economic syndrome" creating an enormous socio-economic and public health burden in poor countries. Obesity has doubled over the past few decades, with 15 percent of children overweight and 25 percent at risk of overweight (Patrick et al. 2005). According to International Obesity Task Force (IOTF), among (5-17) year children, approximately 10 percent children are obese globally though it is unequally distributed with the prevalence ranging from over 30 percent in America to less than 2 percent in Sub-Saharan Africa (Lobstein et al. 2004). The prevalence is 20 percent in UK and Australia, 15.8 percent in Saudi Arabia, 15.6 percent in Thailand, 10 percent in Japan and 7.8 percent in Iran (Al-Nuaim et al. 1996 and Mo-Suwan et al. 1993).

The prevalence behind the childhood obesity may vary according to individual lifestyle and their socio-economic status. Over the past few years, childhood obesity has increased due to changing lifestyle pattern and purchasing junk food, increasing hours of inactivity due addiction of television, videogames which have replaced outdoor games and other activities (Gortmaker et al. 1996; Andersen et al. 1998; Dietz et al. 1985;Rideout et al. 2003; French et al. 2003; Avena et al. 2003). Many researches demonstrate that childhood obesity is associated with many health and psychological problems like – depression, sleep disorders, asthma, and cardiovascular complications and type 2diabetes which are emerging in childhood and later in adult life (Flodmark et al. 2006). Patrick and Nicklas' (2005) review of literature investigates factors behind poor diet and demonstrate how parental factors may impact on children obesity.

Increased duration of TV watching as one of the determinants of obesity was first noticed by Dietz and Gortmaker (1985). TV channels are full of advertisements on foods. These foods may not have much nutritional values. The children consume the advertised goods, including cereals, sweets and salty snacks. Parental feeding style is also important (Birch and Fisher, 1998). Studies demonstrate that adolescents associate junk food with pleasure, independence, convenience whereas liking healthy food is considered odd (Chapman and Maclean, 1993). Study revealed that place of residence and parent education is highly associated with childhood overweight and obesity (Ghosh, 2011).

It is also seen that parental obesity influences the child's obesity because children living with obese parents, especially with obese mother, are more likely to be overweight or obese (Gibson et al. 2007; Wang et al. 2002). Children are more likely to be obese when both parents are obese compared to children with only one of the parents being obese or no one beingobese (Lake et al. 1997). But during childhood, genetic factor accounts for less than 5 per cent for childhood obesity (Anderson et al. 2006).

According to World Bank estimation, India is the highest ranking countries of the world for the number of children suffering from malnutrition. In India, societies are rapidly urbanizing, and lifestyle is changing. There is increase in energy intake through high fat consumption. All these factors result into increase of adult obesity. There is a large disparity of intensity of obesity between rural and urban areas and more so between rich and poor families. This results into high prevalence of obesity among the urban rich (Shetty et al. 1999; Aggarwal et al. 2008 and Raj et al. 2007).

Ramachandran et al. (2002) found that prevalence of overweight is 22.0 percent among the students in better off schools and 4.5 percent among the lower income schools in Chennai. Kapil et al. (2002) found prevalence of overweight among the students in the schools where tuition fee was more than Rs. 2,500 per month, to be 31 per cent including 7.5 percent obese. In Pune, prevalence of overweight children is 24.0 percent in a well-off school and 6.0 percent in a corporation school. In Orissa, the percentage of overweight or obese children is 28.69 percent among (5-9) year aged children (Patnaik et al. 2010). Percentage of overweight (5.10%) was reported to be higher among girls than boys (2.34%) in Manipur (Singh and Devi, 2012). Over-protein and forced feeding by parents, false traditional beliefs about health and nutrition, low knowledge about nutrition in parents and caregivers also contribute to obesity. Again, limited availability of open spaces and parks due to population expansion and illegal settlements with abundance of fast food outlets and eating points increase the chance of the child becoming obese (Kar et al. 2015).

So, it is seen that apart from the socio-economic condition, there may be other factors which influence obesity.In this context, the present study is conducted in one of the urban places in India (Kolkata). The main objectives of the study are (i) to see the prevalence of overweight and obesity among children aged 6-10 years, (ii) to see the relationship of obesity with economic condition and lastly, (iii) to see how far behavioral pattern like duration of TV watching, playing indoor and outdoor games and habit of eating unhealthy junk food items are associated with obesity.

METHODOLOGY

This study is a part of the project which was sanctioned from Planned Budget of Indian Statistical Institute during 2013-2015. This is a micro level cross-section study using stratified sampling scheme. Our population ideally consists of (6-10) year old children in Kolkata Corporation and its peripheral areas. Due to obvious difficulty of identifying the children of proper age-group, we have restricted our study to only school-going children, studying at class I to IV. Total 20 schools are selected randomly for our study. The total study was divided into two phases. All the students of selected schools were included in the first phase of study. Approximately 30 percent of the total children, who were selected in the 1st phase, were considered for detailed study in the second phase.

Due to differentiation of socio-economic background, type of school has been considered as one of the criteria. The reason is that the upper class or more economically affluent people try to admit their children in private school than in public schools. We have restricted our study only to two types of schools – (i) Private and (ii) Public schools. The total number of children in the sample was 5216, of which 2738 were girls and 2478 were boys. Anthropometric measurements such as height and weight were taken from all the students of the selected schools following standard techniques (Weiner and Lourei, 1981). Body mass index (BMI) was calculated by using the formula –Weight (Kg)/Height (mts.)^2. So, BMI for age is used to classify each child into different nutritional status like underweight, normal, overweight and obese for each age and gender. Age and gender specific cut-points as per CDC (Center for Disease Control) where below 5th percentile is considered as underweight, 5th percentile to below 85th percentile for the age and sex is normal, 85th to below 95th percentile is overweight and 95th percentile and above is obese (WHO, 2006).

In the 2nd phase, in each school, all the children (class 1– IV) were divided into two groups according to health status namely 'overweight or obese' and 'non-overweight.' From each school, 40 to 50 from 'obese or overweight' and 40 -50 from 'non-overweight' group were selected randomly for detailed survey. The total sample size in this phase was 1682. Information on the whole day activities of the last seven days on duration of TV watching, time spent for indoor, out-door games and consumption of junk food was taken.The dietary factors that were examined consisted of consumption of fast food, sugary beverages, snack foods though it depends on amount of consumption.

The average duration of one day was calculated from the seven days of these activities. Besides this, information was also taken about the parent's nutritional status and morbidity status of children on non-communicable diseases like thyroid, diabetes or respiratory trouble etc., during the last fifteen days prior to data collection. This was collected based on re-call method from the students or from their respective parents.

Data collection was carried out from September 2013 to October 2014 by a team of trained researchers, which was supported by Indian Statistical Institute.The date of birth of each pupil was taken from the school records and cross checked from their respective parents or guardian. Contact numbers of their parents were collected from the students or from school records or diaries. Other queries, if any, were taken from the guardians of the children directly or through phone.

Descriptive analysis was done for health and nutritional status of children along with some behavioral pattern like duration of TV watching, time spent for indoor and out-door games, consumption of junk food, about parent's nutritional statusand children's morbidity status through percentage variation andmean BMI. For multivariate table analysis, Chi-square tests were done. Categorical Logistic regressions were carried out for nutritional status of children ontype of school and some behavioral pattern to identify the significant factors associated with overweight and obesity. Here, dependent variable was binary with overweight or obese children given value 1 and others 0. Behavioral pattern with different categories were taken as independent variables. The statistical package for the social sciences (SPSS, version 18.0) was used for all the analysis. Significance levels of $p<.01$; 0.05 and 0.1 were considered.

RESULTS

Besides presenting descriptive statistics like percentages, means in the form of multivariate tables, the paper carries out logistic regression to identify the possible risk factors of overweight and obesity among 6 to 10-year children in Kolkata.

Tables 1 & 2 represent the nutritional status of (6-10) year children through body mass index. Here it is seen from the table that out of total 5216 children, 47.50 percent were boys and 52.50 percent were girls. Among the total number of 5216 children, 14.5 percent children were underweight, 53.1 percent were normal, 10.2 percent were overweight, 22.2 percent were obese, and 32.4 percent were overweight (ov) or obese. It is also noticeable that obesity was more among boys than girls.

Table 1. Percentage distribution of nutritional status (BMI forage) of (6-10) year old children in Kolkata

Age (years)	UW	Normal	Overweight	Obese	Overweight & Obese	N
6	14.0	55.8	9.1	23.1	32.2	1030 (100.0)
7	15.1	53.3	9.4	22.2	31.6	1514 (100.0)
8	13.2	53.5	11.0	22.4	33.4	1442 (100.0)
9	14.4	51.6	11.3	22.6	33.9	970 (100.0)
10	21.2	51.9	10.8	16.2	26.9	260 (100.0)
6-10	14.5	53.1	10.2	22.2	32.4	5216 (100.0)

Type of school was considered as one of the layers for stratification of socio-economy. Table 3 shows the nutritional status among the (6-10) year children in public schools in Kolkata. It is seen that in Public school, out of total 3758 children, 14.9percent were underweight, 55.3 percent were normal, 10.2 percent were overweight, 19.7 percent were obese, and 29.8 percent were overweight or obese.

Table 4 presents the same for private schools in Kolkata. In private schools, it is seen that out of 1478 children, 13.5 percent children were underweight, 47.5 percent were normal, 10.4 percent were overweight, 28.6 percent were obese and total 39.0 percent children were overweight or obese.

Table 2. Percentage distribution of nutritional status (BMI for age) of (6-10) year old children in Kolkata by sex

Age (years)	Boys						Girls					
	N	UW	Normal	Overweight	Obese	Overweight & Obese	N	Underweight	Normal	Overweight	Obese	Overweight & obese
6	576 (100.0)	10.8	52.4	10.9	25.9	36.8	454 (100.0)	18.1	55.5	6.8	19.6	26.4
7	716 (100.0)	12.4	50.6	8.4	28.6	37.0	798 (100.0)	17.4	55.8	10.4	16.4	26.8
8	655 (100.0)	11.1	52.7	9.5	26.7	36.2	787 (100.0)	14.9	54.1	12.2	18.8	31.0
9	414 (100.0)	12.1	49.8	8.5	29.7	38.2	556 (100.0)	16.2	53.1	13.5	17.3	30.8
10	117 (100.0)	17.1	50.4	12.0	20.5	32.5	143 (100.0)	24.5	53.1	9.8	12.6	22.4
6-10	2478 (100.0)	11.9	51.4	9.4	27.3	36.7	2738	16.9	54.6	10.9	17.6	28.5

Table 3. Percentage distribution of nutritional status (BMI for age) of (6-10) year old children in public schools in Kolkata

Age (years)	N	UW	Normal	Overweight	Obese	Overweight & Obese
6	779 (100.0)	13.6	56.5	8.7	21.2	29.9
7	1141 (100.0)	14.3	55.7	9.7	20.2	30.0
8	1079 (100.0)	15.0	54.9	11.2	18.9	30.1
9	621 (100.0)	15.9	53.6	11.3	19.2	30.4
10	118 (100.0)	22.9	55.1	8.5	13.6	22.0
6-10	3758 (100.0)	14.9	55.3	10.2	19.7	29.8

Table 4. Percentage distribution of nutritional status (BMI for age) of (6-10) year old children in Private schools in Kolkata

Age (years)	N	UW	Normal	Overweight	Obese	Overweight & Obese
6	251 (100.0)	15.1	45.4	10.4	29.1	39.4
7	373 (100.0)	17.4	45.8	8.6	28.2	36.7
8	363 (100.0)	7.7	49.3	10.2	32.8	43.0
9	349 (100.0)	11.7	48.1	11.5	28.7	40.1
10	142 (100.0)	19.7	49.3	12.7	18.3	31.0
6-10	1478 (100.0)	13.5	47.5	10.4	28.6	39.0

Table 5 describes the differences of obesity between public and private schools in Kolkata. It is seen that obesity was unanimously higher in private schools than public schools among (6-10) year children. The magnitudes of differences between boys and girls show that it was the highest among the boys and the lowest among the girls.

Table 5. Percentagedifferences of obesities between two types of school of (6-10) year oldchildren in Kolkata

Age	Total				Boys				Girls			
	Public school (x)	Private school (y)	Differences (y-x)	% of differences (y-x)/x *100	Public school (x)	Private school (y)	Differences (y-x)	% of differences (y-x)/x *100	Public school (x)	Private school (y)	Differences (y-x)	% of differences (y-x)/x *100
6	29.9	39.4	9.5	31.77	35.2	41.2	6.0	17.04	23.6	36.7	13.1	55.51
7	30.0	36.7	6.7	22.33	33.8	46.0	12.2	36.09	26.7	27.2	0.5	1.87
8	30.1	43.0	12.9	42.85	30.1	50.0	19.9	66.11	30.1	34.4	4.3	14.28
9	30.4	40.1	9.7	31.90	31.1	46.2	15.1	48.55	30.2	32.5	2.3	7.61
10	22.0	31.0	9.0	40.90	11.8	41.0	29.2	247.45	26.2	16.9	-9.3	-35.41
6-10	29.8	39.0	9.2	30.87	32.3	45.6	13.	40.24	27.8	30.7	2.9	10.43

Table 6. Relationship between different independent variables with normal, overweight or obese children of total and by gender differences in Kolkata

Name of the variables	Total				Boys				Girls			
	N	Others	OV & obese	Chi-square	N	Others	OV & obese	Chi-square	N	Others	OV & obese	Chi-square
Type of school				3.843 df = 1				4.062 df = 1				0.433 df = 1
Public	1303	54.3	45.7	0.050	573	55.5	44.5	0.044	730	53.3	46.7	0.510
Private	379	48.5	51.5		302	48.3	51.7		77	49.4	50.6	
Daily Av. Durationof TV watching												
No	150	60.0	40.0	10.282	63	63.5	36.5	9.514	87	57.5	42.5	3.333
< 1- < 3	1146	54.2	45.8	df = 3	606	54.8	45.2	df = 3	540	53.5	46.5	df = 3
3- < 4	190	47.4	52.6	0.016	111	43.2	56.8	0.023	79	53.2	46.8	0.343
4 & above	189	45.5	54.5		91	46.2	53.8		98	44.9	55.1	
Daily Av. duration on Spending on indoor games												
0	432	55.1	44.9	1.509	282	57.1	42.9	3.736	150	51.3	48.7	1.031
>0 - < 2	1159	52.2	47.8	df = 2	556	51.6	48.4	df = 2	603	52.7	47.3	df = 2
2 or more	91	52.7	47.3	0.589	37	43.2	56.8	0.154	54	59.3	40.7	0.597
Daily Av. duration on Spending on outdoor games												
0	638	46.1	53.9	19.812	279	47.0	53.0	6.070	359	45.4	54.6	16.352
>0 - < 2	967	57.0	43.0	df = 2	535	55.9	44.1	df = 2	432	58.3	41.7	df = 2
2 or more	77	59.7	40.3	0.000	61	55.7	44.3	0.048	16	75.0	25.0	0.000
Daily having av. junk food items												
No	68	47.1	52.9	6.983	26	42.3	57.7	5.155	42	50.0	50.0	2.544
Average (1-6 items)	1455	54.2	45.8	df = 2 0.030	729	54.7	45.3	df = 2 0.076	726	53.7	46.3	df = 2 0.280
Heavy (7-8 items)	159	44.0	56.0		120	45.0	55.0		39	41.0	59.0	
Whether Mother is obese												
No	1142	56.6	43.4	18.154	582	56.9	43.1	10.312	560	56.2	43.8	7.887
Yes	539	45.5	54.5	df = 1 0.000	293	45.4	54.6	df = 1 0.001	246	45.5	54.5	df = 1 0.005
Whether Father is obese												
No	1186	55.8	44.2	14.239	608	55.8	44.2	6.468	578	55.9	44.1	7.900
Yes	482	45.6	54.4	df = 1 0.000	263	46.4	53.6	df = 1 0.011	219	44.7	55.3	df = 1 0.005
Whether Parents' are obese												
No	1480	54.9	45.1	22.249	769	55.1	44.9	12.860	711	54.7	45.3	9.431
Yes	188	36.7	63.3	df = 1 0.000	102	36.3	63.7	df = 1 0.000	86	37.2	62.8	df = 1 0.002

Table 6. (Continued)

Name of the variables	Total				Boys				Girls			
	N	Others	OV & obese	Chi-square	N	Others	OV & obese	Chi-square	N	Others	OV & obese	Chi-square
Morbidity												
No diseases	1514	53.7	46.3	7.147 df = 2 0.025	809	53.2	46.8	3.417 df = 2 0.181	705	54.3	45.7	5.263 df = 2 0.072
Thyroid or Diabetes	19	26.3	73.7		9	22.2	77.8		10	30.0	70.0	
Respiratory or others	143	47.6	52.4		53	52.8	47.2		90	44.4	55.6	

Table 6 summarizes the level of association between overweight or obesity of children with type of school and some behavioral patterns like duration of TV watching, indoor and outdoor games, heredity and non-communicable morbidity among total children and by gender differences. It is seen that children of private school were more obese than public school. It is also seen that obesity has direct relationship with duration of TV watching, heavy amount of junk food items (at least more than seven items), mother's and father's individual obesity as well as parental obesity and suffering from diseases by thyroid or diabetes. All these results were statistically significance at 1% level of significant. Outdoor games had only negative effect on obesity and it was also statistically significant at 1% or 5% level of significant.

Table 7 is showing the association of (6-10) year children's obesity with different independent variables through categorical logistic regression analysis. Here nutritional status was the dependent variable which was regressed on different independent variables. Analysis revealed that children of private school students were always more overweight or obese than those of public school and the result were statistically significant at 5% level of significance among all children and among boys. Duration of TV watching above 3 or more hours, having junk food items above 7 per week, individual parental obesity and victims of thyroid or diabetes had significant impact on increasing obesity among total children and among boys. In case of girls, only parent's individual obesity and thyroid or diabetes sufferers had significant impact on increasing obesity. It is also seen that duration of outdoor games was significantly negatively related to obesity among the children as well as separately among boys and girls.

Table 7. Results of categorical logistic regressions of obesity with different socio-economic variables among (6-10) year old children in Kolkata

Name of the variables	Total	Boys	Girls
Type of school			
Public®	1.00	1.00	1.00
Private	1.729*	1.359*	1.090
Daily Average durationof TV watching			
No®	1.00	1.00	1.00
< 1- < 3	1.170	1.441	1.026
3- < 4	1.492*	2.079*	1.089
4 & above	1.626*	1.964*	1.491
Daily Average duration on Spending on indoor games (hrs.)			
0.0®	1.00	1.00	1.00
>0.0 - < 2.0	1.076	1.267	0.805
2.0 or more	0.978	1.369	0.676
Daily Average duration on spending on outdoor games (hrs.)			
0.0®	1.00	1.00	1.00
>0.0 - < 2.0	0.650**	0.715*	0.586**
2.0 or more	0.507**	0.623	0.264*
Daily having of average junk food items			
Average (1-6 items) ®	1.00	1.00	1.00
No junk food	1.188	1.203	1.168
Heavy (7-8 items)	1.543*	1.537*	1.610
Whether Mother is obese			
No®	1.00	1.00	1.00
Yes	1.405**	1.408*	1.427*
Whether Father is obese			
No®	1.00	1.00	1.00
Yes	1.350*	1.278	1.502*
Whether parents are obese			
No®	1.00	1.00	1.00
Yes	1.226	1.260	1.048
Morbidity			
No diseases®	1.00	1.00	1.00
Thyroid or Diabetes	3.895*	5.158*	3.041
Respiratory or others	1.330	1.073	1.526*

*® = Reference category; ** p < 0.01; *p < 0.05.

Discussion and Conclusion

India is a fast-growing economy, currently undergoing major epidemiological, nutritional and demographic transitions. These transitions tend to promote obesity in all age groups. Here, the aim of the study was to estimate the prevalence of overweight or obesity among 6 to 10 years children in Kolkata and to see the various associative contributing factors on obesity like socio-economic group, lifestyle, diet and family history of the children. The study was done among 5216 children from 20 different schools in greater Kolkata. Among them, 52.5 percent (2738) were girls and 47.5 percent (2478) were boys. Also, 14.5 percent children were underweight, 53.1 percent were normal, 10.2 percent were overweight, 22.2 percent were obese, and 32.4 percent were overweight (ov) or obese. It is also seen that 36.7 percent boys and 28.5 percent girls were overweight or obese. So, it is obvious that obesity was more among boys than girls. To assess in an indirect way to find out the relationship between obesity with different socio-economy, firstly, the students were selected from two types of schools like public and private schools. The reason is that the upper class or more economically affluent people try to admit their child or children in private schools than public schools. It is seen that in public schools, 29.8 percent children were overweight & obese and in private schools, 39.0 percent children were overweight or obese.

Besides socio-economy, we have considered other factors which influenceobesity directly or indirectly. Among these, TV watching was presumed to be one of the most important target factors. We wanted to see how far TV watching influences the increaseof obesity among childrenbecause in the 21st century, good friends or bad friends have been replaced at home by media like Television, mobile etc. It is also seen from our study that only 9 percent students were not watching TV. About 68 percent to 69 percent children were watching TV one hour to less than three hours.It is seen that duration of TV watching was directly related with obesity and the result is statistically significant at 1% level of significance. Sports and exercises have been replaced by the habit of TV watching is reducing metabolism. Besides TV watching, it is seen that duration of indoor games were directly related with the obesity and outdoor games was negatively related with obesity because those children who played daily on the average less than twohours in a week are more obese than who played more than twohours. These studies were consistent with previous studies in different countries (Hernaandez et al. 1999; Ross et al. 1998; Tremblay et al. 2003 and Prentice et al. 1995).

Let us now focus our attention to the consumption of junk food and chocolate. It is seen that junk food items andchocolates had direct impacts on obesity because the children who consumed daily more than 6 items on the average are more obese than the other group. Generally, junk food (bakery items, pizza, burger, cheese, butter, oily items, chocolate) intake tended to be more common among overweight and obese children than normal children (Klesges et al. 1995; Wolfe et al. 1994). And this food items had more fat than protein and carbohydrate and fat is stored more efficiently than carbohydrates or proteins which finally results in obesity or overweight (Birch et al. 1998; Rolls et al. 1994; Blundell et al. 1993 and Poppitt, 1995). Obesity may also be hereditary because it is seen from our study that lowest percentage of overweightor obese children were found among the non-obese parents and the highest percentage were found among the obese parents.

Obesity among (6-10) year children is increasing in an alarming rate in Kolkata. In general, 32.4 percent of (6-10) year children fall in the category of overweight or obese. Our study also confirms that the children of private schools were significantly more obese compared to public schools which indirectly reflects the socio-economic conditions that affects the children's health status. Besides, it is seen that duration of Television watching, duration of out-door playing; habits of junk food item which were very much responsible for increasing the obesity. It is also seen that certain non-communicable diseases like diabetes or thyroid were more prevalent among the obese children than normal children. And those children having family history of obesity were more likely to become obese or overweightand had a high chance of suffering from thyroid or diabetes.

So, in conclusion, it can be said that the rising rate of childhood obesity is one of the most significant problems that we are facing in our society. The children are becoming more attracted to TV watching and indoor games which are associated with least physical exercise. So, intervention of activitiesmust be conducted in the community and as well as in school premisesfor preventing overweight or obesity. Moreover, parents must be aware and taking some effective actionsat an early stage of life of their childrenat home.

REFERENCES

Aggarwal T, Bhatia RC, Singh D, Sobti PC. 2008. Prevalence of obesity and overweight in affluent adolescents from Ludhiana, Punjab.*Indian Pediatr.*45:500–502.

Al-Nuaim AR, Bamgboye EA, al-Herbish A. 1996. The pattern of growth and obesity in Saudi Arabian male school children. I*nternationalJournal of Obesity and Related Metabolic Disorders*. 20:1000-1005.

Anderson RE, Crespo CJ, Bartleh SJ, Cheskin LJ, Pratt MM. 1998. Relationship of physical activity and television watching with body weight and level of fatness among children. *JAMA*. 279:938-942.

Anderson PM, Butcher KE. 2006. Childhood obesity: Trends and potential causes. *Future Child.* 16:19-45.

Avena NM, Hoebel BG. 2003. A diet promoting sugar dependency causes behavioral cross-sensitization to a low dose of amphetamine. *Neuroscience*.122:17–20.

Birch LL, Fisher JO. 1998. Development of eating behaviors among children and adolescents. *Pediatrics*. 101:539-549.

Blundell JE, Burley VJ, Cotton JR, Lawton CL. 1993. Dietary fat and the control of energy intake: evaluating the effects of fat on meal size and post meal satiety. *Am J ClinNutr*. 57:772s-778s.

Chapman G, Maclean H. 1993. "Junk food" and "healthy food": meaning of food in adolescent women's culture. *Journal of Nutrition Educationand Behaviour*.25:108- 113.

Center for Disease Control and Prevention.*Contributing factors*. 2010. (Available from: http://w.w.w.cdc.gov//obesity/childhood/contributing factors.htm).

Davison KK, Birch LL. 2001. Childhood overweight: A contextual model and recommendations for future research. *Obesity Review*. 2(3):159–171.

Dietz W, Gortmaker S. 1985. Do we fatten our children at the TV set? Obesity and television viewing in children and adolescents. *Pediatrics*. 75: 807-812.

Freedman DS, Kettel Khan L, Serdula MK, Dietz WH et al. 2005.The relation of childhood BMI to adult adiposity: the Bogalusa Heart Study. *Pediatrics*. 115:22-27.

Flodmark C, Marucs C, Britton M. (2006). Interventions to prevent obesity in children and adolescents: a systemic literature review. *International Journal of Obesity*. 30:579-589.

French SA, Lin BH, Guthrie JF. 2003. National trends in soft drink consumption among children and adolescents age 6 to 17 years: Prevalence, amounts, and sources, 1977/1978 to 1994/1998. *J Am Diet Assoc*.103(10):1326–1331.

Ghosh A. 2011.Rural–Urban Comparison in Prevalence of Overweight and Obesity among Children and Adolescents of Asian Indian Origin. *Asia Pacific Journal of Public Health*. 23(6):928 – 935.

Gibson LY, Byrne SM, Davis EA, Blair E, Jacoby P, Zubrick SR. 2007.The role of family and maternal factors in childhood obesity. *Medical Journal of Australia*. 186:591 595

Gortmaker S, Must A, Sobal A, Peterson K, Colditz S, Dietz W, 1996.Television viewing as a cause of increasing obesity among children in United States, 1986- 1990. *Archives of Pediatrics and Adolescent Medicine*. 150:356-362.

Hernaandez B, gortmaker SL, Colditz GA, Peterson KE, Laird NM, Parra-Cabera S. 1999. Association of obesity with physical activity, television programs and other forms of video viewing among children in Mexico City. *Int J Obesity*. 23:845-854.

Hill JO, Peters JC. 1998. Environmental contributions to the obesity epidemic. *Science*. 280:1371–1374.

Kapil U, Singh P, Pathak P, Dwivedi SN, Bhasin S. 2002. Prevalence of obesity amongst affluent adolescent schoolgirls in Chennai in 1981 & 1998. *Indian Pediatr*. 39:449-452.

Kar SS. 2015. Prevention of childhood obesity in India. *Journal of NaturalScience, Biology and Medicine*. 6(1):12-17.

Klesges RC, Klesges LM, ECK LH, Shelton ML. 1995.A longitudinal analysis of accelerated weight gain in preschool children. *Pediatrics*. 95:126-130.

Lake JK, Power C, Cole TJ.1997. Child to adult body mass index in the 1958 British birth cohort: associations with parental obesity. *Arch Dis Child*.77: 376–381.

Lobstein T, Baur L, Uauy R. 2004. *Obesity in children and young people: A crisis in public health. Report to the WHO*. Published by IASO International Obesity Task Force, London.

Mo-Suwan L, Junjana C, Puetapaiboon A. 1993.Increasing obesity in school children in transitional society and the effect of the weight control programme. *South East Asian journal of Tropical Medicine and Public Health*. 24: 590-594.

Patric H, Nicklas T. 2005. A review of family and social determinant of children's eating patterns and diet quality. *Journals of the American College of Nutrition*. 24:83-92.

Patnaik S, Patnaik L, Patnaik S, Hussain M. 2010. Prevalence of overweight and obesity in a private school of Orissa, India. *The Internet Journal of Epidemiology*. 10: 1-9.

Poppit SD. 1995. Energy density of diets and obesity. *Int. J Obes*. 19: S20-S26.

Prentice AM, Jebb SA. 1995. Obesity in Britain: Gluttonyor Sloth? *BMJ*. 311:437-439.

Raj M, Sundaram KR, Paul M, Deepa AS, Kumar RK. 2007. Obesity in Indian children: time trends and relationship with hypertension. *Natl Med J India*. 20:288-293.

Ramachandran A, Snehalatha C, Vinitha R, Megha T, Sathish Kumar CK, Sheeba L, Joseph S, Vijaya V. 2002. Prevalence of overweight in urban Indian adolescent school children. *Diabetes Res ClinPract*. 57:185-190.

Rideout VJ, Vandewater EA, Wartella EA. 2003.*Zero to Six: Electronic Media in the Lives of Infants, Toddlers and Preschoolers*. Menlo Park, CA: Henry J. Kaiser Family Foundation.

Rolls BJ, Kim-Harris S, Fischman MW, Foltin RW, Moran TH, Stoner SA. 1994. Satiety after preloads with different amounts of fat and carbohydrate: implications for obesity. *Am J ClinNutr*. 60:476-487.

Ross EA, Carlos JC, Susan JB, Lawrence JC, Michael P. 1998. Relationship of physical activity and television watching with Body weight and level of fatness among children. *JAMA*. 279:938-942.

Rossener S. 2002. Obesity the disease of twenty-first century. *International Journal of Obesity*. 26: 52-54.

Shetty PS. 1999. Obesity in children in developing societies: indicator of economic progress or a prelude to a health disaster. *Indian Pediatr*. 36:11-15.

Singh MS, Devi RKN. 2012. Nutritional Status among the Urban Meitei Children and Adolescents of Manipur, Northeast India. *Journal of Anthropology*. 2013:1-5.

Styne DM. 2001. Childhood and adolescent obesity: Prevalence and significance. *Pediatric Clinics of North America*. 48: 823-854.

Tremblay MS, Willms JD. 2003. Is the Canadian childhood obesity epidemic related to physical inactivity? *Int J Obesity*. 27:1100-1105.

Wang Y, Lobstein T. 2006. Worldwide trends in childhood overweight and obesity. *Int.J. Pediatr. Obese*. 1:11-25.

Weiner JS, Lourie JA. 1981. *Practical Human Biology*. Academic Press. New York.

Wolfe WS, Campbell CC, Frongillo JR EA, Hass JD, Meinik TA. 1994. Overweight School children in New York State: Prevalence and characteristics. *Am J Public Health*. 84: 807-813.

World Health Organization Multicentre Growth Reference Study Group. 2006. *WHO Child growth standards: length/height for age, weight for age, weight for length, weight for height and body mass index for age methods and development*. Geneva: WHO.

In: Contemporary Issues in Childhood … ISBN: 978-1-53617-348-2
Editors: J. Ratan Ghosh and K. Bose

Chapter 8

SOCIAL ECONOMIC STATUS IS ASSOCIATED WITH NUTRITIONAL STATUS OF CHILDREN IN WEST SUMATRA, INDONESIA

Nur Indrawaty Lipoeto[1,*] and Helmizar[2]
[1]Department of Nutrition, Faculty of Medicine,
Andalas University, Padang, Indonesia
[2]Department of Nutrition, Faculty of Public Health,
Andalas University, Padang, Indonesia

ABSTRACT

Nutritional status is a strong indicator that can be used to show the level of social and economic development of a country. Several classical studies by Martorell (1986) and Tanner et al., (1982) conducted in various countries have shown that there are differences in average height and growth rates that differ between children from poor families compared to children from rich families in the same nation. If the difference in growth of rich family children is caused by genetic factors is 2-3 cm, the difference caused by the economic unequal gap in the same nation is around 10-12

* Corresponding Author's Email: indra.liputo@gmail.com.

cm. In studies comparing the growth rates of various nations, it was found that children from rich families in nations in Latin America, Africa, and India, had growth rates that were not different from those of European families. Whereas in Asian children, genetic differences still play an important role, Asian children experience better growth in line with secular trends but their optimal growth potential is still lower than the average growth. This difference is more evident after children reach puberty. Mortorell (1986) and Tanner (1982) has become the basis of various studies that prove the relationship between height and economic status. A report from Ghana by Hong (2007) shows that children at the lowest socioeconomic status of 20% in their community have a double risk of suffering stunting from the richest 20% in the same area and this result was not controlled by age, gender, order of children in the family, length of breastfeeding, birth weight, age at delivery, body mass index, education, access to clean water, toilet washing facilities, residence, and geographical area. Furthermore, a study in Angola (Kennedy et al., 2005) shows that at the same economic level there was no difference in the prevalence of stunting both in rural and urban areas.

Stunting during the early period of life is critical, because the first few years in life are a particularly important period in human development. The development of cognitive abilities begins in this period (Mendez and Adair, 1999; Grantham Mcgregor, 2007). Stunting during infancy and early childhood adversely affects cognitive development. Crookston et al., (2010) found that stunted children aged 6 and 18 months, and were followed up at age 4.5 to 6 years old, have had lower intellectual ability than children who were not stunted. Kar et al., (2008) conducted a study on children aged 5-7 years and found significant differences in cognitive development between stunted children and non-stunted children. A study in Vietnam reported an increase by a standard deviation in height for age Z score (HAZ) leads to an increase by one fourth of a standard deviation of the log score of language ability (Le Thuc Duc, 2009). These were previously confirmed by other studies (Mendez M. A. and Adair L. S., 1999; Walker S. P. et al., 2005; Grantham McGregor et al., 2007, Grantham Mcgregor, S., 2007).

Psychosocial stimulation in early childhood had significant benefits in the improvement of stunted children's psychological development. Stunted children who received stimulation had levels of anxiety, depressive syndrome, and self esteem similar to those of the nonstunted children (Walker S. P. et al., 2006). Maternal role is the key in providing psychosocial stimulation. Improvement of maternal education will increase the possibility of catch-up growth and levels of cognition in later adolescence (Crookston et al., 2010).

This paper describes a study conducted in West Sumatra, Indonesia. The study was done to determine the relationship between socio-economic statuses and nutritional status.

METHODS

The study was conducted in two sub-districts in Padang, capital city of West Sumatra Province in Indonesia. The population was new children enrolled in primary schools. The sample was first grade children and as many as 124 people in selected elementary schools, which was selected through a multistage random sampling. Subdistricts were divided into urban and suburban. Of the 5 sub-districts in the urban setting, North of Padang Utara was chosen. Of the 6 suburban settings, Pauh was chosen. Two elementary schools in Padang Utara were selected and three elementary schools in Pauh were selected for this study. All first grade pupils and their mothers from selected schools were included in the study with exclusive criterias: twins, having physical disabilities, living outside the research area, absent during the study and mothers who are not willing to be interviewed and who are not found at the time of data collection.

All children recieved anthropometric measurements for weight and height assessments. Mothers were interviewed to assess socioeconomic status, family characteristics, and accessibility level of health services and sanitation facilities. Height was measured by using microtoise that has an accuracy up to 0.1 cm.

Data was analysed using SPSS 20.0. To find out the relationship between socio-economic status and nutritional status, chi -square test was used with significancy level of p value <0.05. Pair t test and Pearson correlation were also used.

RESULTS

A total of 153 subjects were eligible in the study but only 80% of all first grade students were included in this study due to absence, living outside the study area, and mothers were not found during home visits.

Characteristics of the Subjects

First grade students in urban areas were relatively younger than first class students in the suburban, with significant differences. The average age of children in both locations is 6.8 years. Mother's age in the urban and in the suburban was similar which was around 51-54% less or equal to 35 years. Mothers in urban areas had higher education; 86% finished high school education or higher. Only 24% of mothers in the suburban area did the same.

Socioeconomic status was measured by using total expenditure per capita per month, amount of food expenditure per capita per month, and percentage of expenditure per capita for food every month. The average total expenditure per capita was higher in urban areas compared to the suburban areas. The average expenditure for food in the urban was 2 times higher than the average amount in the suburban. The percentage of food expenditure in urban areas ranges from 22-27% of total expenditure while in the suburban was even higher, between 37-87%.

Nutritional Status

The average height of children in urban areas was higher than children in the suburban. Boys in urban areas are 3 cm taller than boys in suburban, as shown in Table 1.

The range of boys' height in urban areas was 109.1-129.5 cm and in the suburban was 103.3-118.4 cm. The range of height of first grade girls in urban girls was 108.7-126.2 cm and in the suburban was 104.0-126.0 cm. The statistical test results of the differences between these two groups were very significant ($p = 0.000025$).

The tallest children from the high expenditure group was 10.1 cm taller than children from lower expenditure in urban area, whereas in suburban, the difference was 6.1 cm. Children from families with low food expenditure in urban areas are 4.1 cm taller than their peers in the same group in the suburban, while children with high expenditures in urban were 2.9 cm taller with their peers in the suburban.

Table 1. Differences of nutritional status and height based on gender and expenditure between urban and suburban

Characteristics	Urban	Suburban	p
Height: Boys	115.9 ± 4.3	112.8 ± 4.6	<0.01
Girls	116.8 ± 3.7	111.6 ± 4.3	<0.0001
High total expend	116.4 ± 4.10	116.1 (± 3.21)	<0.05
Low total expend	112.0 ± 5.72)	112.4 (± 3.79)	<0.05
	p < 0.001	p < 0.001	
High food expend	116.5 ± 4.23	113.6 ± 3.53	<0.001
Low food expend	116.0 ± 4.14	111.9 ± 5.59	<0.001
	p < 0.05	p < 0.05	
Stunting	7 (10.0%)	28 (51.9%)	<0.0001
Normal	63 (90.0%)	26 (48.1%)	

Pearson correlation tests were also done between various indicators of socio-economic status with nutritional status. We found that there was close relationship between economic status and height. Total expenditure, food expenditure, and percentage of food expenditure had a positive linear relationship with height of the children.

DISCUSSION

Total expenditure is a proxy for family socio-economic indicators. In this study, total expenditure per capita per month, total food expenditure and, percentage of food expenditure is significantly lower in suburban families. This is a general description of the situation in developing countries. In India, Venkaiah et al., (2002) reported that 37% of the population in rural areas had poor economic status.

This study reported height differences of children according to gender and location. Boys in urban areas were 3 cm higher compared those in suburban areas while in girls the differences was 5 cm. Girls in urban areas were taller than boys, however, boys were taller than girls in suburban areas. Ulukanligil et al., (2004) found also that boys in school children in urban areas in Turkey are smaller than girls. Moreover, we found that the tallest boy in urban areas was 11 cm higher than the shortest boy in the suburban area, while the tallest girl in the suburban area was 4 cm shorter than the shortest girl in urban areas. The result of this study was similar with the findings of Hakeem (2001) that showed the better the economic status, the fewer children in the short category. Jalal and Soekirman (1990) concluded that the difference in the growth of children from rich families compared to poor families in the same nation was 10-12 cm.

This study found that the prevalence of stunting in children in suburban areas was 51.9%, compared to 10% in urban areas. Ministry of Health of Indonesia, which conducted periodic Basic Health Surveys, reported that the prevalence of stunting in Indonesia was 36.8%, 35.6% and 37.2% between 2007, 2010 and 2013. Ministry of Health of Indonesia also reported the prevalence of stunting children from families in quintile 1-2 was 41.2% compared to only 27.8% in children from quintile 4-5. The result of this study found that there was a significant difference in the relationship between total food expenditure and percentage of food expenditure with height of the children.

Several determinants, such as distribution of income and nutritional status during infancy, are reported to affect the height of children after they reach pre-adolescence (Thomas and Frakenberg, 2002). Stunting is related with duration of education, improvement in body height, and prolongs the number of classes passed, which means higher levels of education (Alderman et al., 2006). Research in Turkey, Ghana and, Bangladesh also consistently reported a close relationship between the socio-economic level and stunting (Turan et al., 2007; Wamani et al., 2006; Pryer et al., 2003). A study in Mexico by Fernald and Neufeld (2007) showed a relationship between stunting and obesity in children from low socioeconomic levels, mothers with low and short education, numbers of children, and low city mastery. Furthermore, the study by Ulukanligil et al., (2004), which examined differences in height of children living in slums and children living in apartments in urban areas in Turkey, showed that the prevalence of stunting in children living in slums was higher than children living in apartments. However, studies in Trinidad and Tobago reported that ethnicity, parental height, birth weight, maternal age at delivery, and number of children in the family were associated with height, while economic status was not related (Rona et al., 2004).

This study supported other studies in other developing countries that shows anthropometric index as a strong indicator of growth of children. The use of the anthropometric index as socio-economic indicator is no doubt. The growth of children in achieving optimal growth potential is the result of adequate nutritional needs. This situation can only be achieved if the socio-economic conditions are getting better and more evenly distributed.

REFERENCES

Alderman H., Hoddinott J., Kinsey B., Longterms of consequences for early childhood malnutrition; *Oxford Economic Papers* 58 (2006); 450-476.

Central Bureau of Statistics. *Results of the 1999-2000 National Socio-Economic Survey (SUSE NAS) in West Sumatra.*

Department of health RI. *1999/2000 TBABS Monitoring Guidelines. Jakarta*, Ministry of Health RI. 1999.

Djumadias A., et al., *Nutritional Status of New Children Entering Elementary School as Population Socio-Economic Indicators.* Jakarta, Nutrition Research Center-Minister of Environment, Ministry of Environment, 1987.

Fernald L. C. and Neufeld L. M., Overweight with concurrent stunting in very child from rural Mexico: prevalence and associated factors. *European Journal of Clinical Nutrition* (2007) 61, 623-632.

Helen Keler Internasional (HKI) Indonesia. *Report on the results of the Nutrition and Health Monitoring Survey in West Sumatra.* Padang. MOH HKI FK. Unand 2000.

Hong R. Effect of Economic Inequalityon Chronic childhood malnutrition in Ghana. *Public Health Nutrition* 2007, 10 (4), 371-378.

Jalal F. Soekirman. Utilization of Anthropometry as an Socio-Economic Indicator. Jakarta. *Indonesian Nutrition.* 1990, 14 (2): 25-36.

Kennedy G., Nantel G., Brouwer I. D., Kok F. J.; Does living in an urban environment converge for childhood nutritional status? Analysis of disparities in nutritional status by wealth and residence in Angola Central African Republic and Senegal; *Public Health Nutrition* 2005, 9 (2), 187-193.

Kodyat B. Completion of Poor Nutrition Problems. Jakarta: *Proceedings of Widyakarya Nasional VI.* 1999.

Martorell R. and Habicht J. P. Growth in Early Childhood in Developing Countries. In: *Human Growth: A comprehensive Tratise*, 2nd Ed. Falner & Tanner (eds). New York: Plenum Publication, 1986.

Pryer J. A., Rogers S., Rahman A., The epidemiology of good nutritional status among children from population with a high prevalence of malnutrition. *Public Health Nutrition* 2003, 7 (2), 311-317.

Simanjuntak G. Height Measurement of New Children Entering School in Sekayam District, West Kalimantan. Jakarta: 1995. *Mirror of the Medical World* No. 01. 24-31.

Soetjiningsih. *Child Development.* Jakarta: EGC. 1995.

Tanner J. M., Hayashi T., Preece M. A., and Cameron. Increase length of leg relative to trunk in Japanese children and adults from 1957 to 1977: Comparison with British and Japanese Americans. *Ann Hum Biol* 1982, 9: 411-423.

Thomas D. and Frakenberg E., Health, nutrition and prosperity: a microeconomic perspective. *World Health Organization Bulletin of World Health Organization* (2002). 80.2. 106.

Turan A., Bereket A., Furman A. et al., The effect of economic status on height, insulin like growth factor (IGF) and IGF binding protein-3 concentration in healthy Turkish children. *European Journal of Clinical Nutrition* (2007) 61. 752-758.

Ulukanligil A., Seyrek A. Anthropomeric status, anemia and intestinal helmintic infections in shantytown and apartment school children in the Sanliurfa Province of Turkey; *European Journal of Clinical Nutrition* (2004) 58; 1056-1061.

Venkaiah K., Damayanti K., Nayak M. U., Vijayaraghavan K., Diet and nutritional status of rural adolescents in India. *European Journal of Clinical Nutrition* (2002) 56; 1119-1125.

Wamani H., Astrom A. N., Peterson R. et al., Predictors of poor anthropometric status among children under 2 years of age in rural Uganda; *Public Health Nutrition* (2006) 9 (3); 320-326.

In: Contemporary Issues in Childhood … ISBN: 978-1-53617-348-2
Editors: J. Ratan Ghosh and K. Bose

Chapter 9

NUTRITIONAL STATUS OF TRIBAL CHILDREN UNDER 5 YEARS OF AGE IN ITDA PADERU DIVISION, ANDHRA PRADESH

***Sunita Sreegiri*[1] *and M. Siva Durga Prasad Nayak*[2,*]**
[1]Department of Community Medicine,
Andhra Medical College/NTRHUS, Gunadala,
Vijayawada, Andhra Pradesh, India
[2]Department of Community Medicine,
RIMS Medical College/NTRHUS, Ongole, Andhra Pradesh, India

ABSTRACT

Nutritional status of any community is influenced by interplay of various factors including beliefs, customs, food availability in the region. Children from tribal groups are particularly under privileged. They have higher rates of morbidity and are known to receive less than desired nutritional intake.

* Corresponding Author's Email: sivadurgaprasadnayak@gmail.com.

The present study was conducted with the objectives to study the feeding practices of Tribal Children aged 6 months to 5 years and to assess the nutritional status of these children.

A Community based cross-sectional study conducted in ITDA Paderu division of Visakhapatnam district. Study population include tribal children in the age group of 6 months to 5 years. A sample of 181 children were surveyed. After taking consent, information was obtained from mother/care taker on feeding practices according to IYCF and IMNCI guidelines.

Majority (88.4%) of children received exclusive breast feeding. In 26% children introduction of solid and semisolid food was delayed beyond 6 months. Among the children aged 6 months to 2 years, 80% had minimum diversity in their diet, 71.2 % had minimum meal frequency and 48.5% were taking minimum acceptable diet. Among the children 2 to 5 years of age, 62.6% were taking 3 meals and 2 nutritious foods per day. Prevalence of Underweight (< -2 of WHO Z score) was found as 49.2%, stunting as 51% and wasting as 32.2%.

Feeding practices of tribal children in the early infancy are satisfactory. However in the late infancy and early childhood, there is deficiency in the frequency and adequacy of the feeds leading to wasting and stunting.

Keywords: Feeding practices, IYCF, Nutritional status, Tribal children, Under 5 children

INTRODUCTION

Nutritional status of any community is influenced by interplay of various factors including beliefs, customs, food availability in the region. This in turn influences the physical growth and nutritional status of the whole community (Varadarajan and Prasad 2009). According to the 2011 census, the scheduled tribes comprise about 8.6% of total India's population (Ministry of Tribal Affairs 2013). Since most of the tribal habitations are located in isolated villages and hamlets coinciding with forest areas, there are natural hurdles in their ability to access nutritious food and also health care. The literacy, economic and health indicators for tribal people are poorer than for the rest of the population which in turn influence their food intake. Women and children from these groups are particularly under privileged. They have higher rates of morbidity, and are known to receive less than desired nutritional intake. According to NFHS-3, 54.5 % children under 5 years belonging to Scheduled Tribes have been reported to be underweight (Ministry of Women and Child development 2011).

METHODOLGY

A Community based cross-sectional study was conducted in ITDA Paderu division of Visakhapatnam district with two objectives viz., To study the feeding practices of Tribal Children aged 6 months to 5 years and to assess the nutritional status of these children. A sample of 181 children (calculated based on prevalence as reported by NNMB study) between 6 months to 5 years was surveyed. Multistage simple random sampling technique was applied to select 9 villages in tribal mandals located in 3 Community Health and Nutrition Centres. A house to house survey was conducted to interview 20 children in each village. In case of less populated villages/ small hamlets, where 20 children could not be covered, the subsequent village/hamlet was included. After taking consent, information was obtained from mother/care taker (above 15 years of age) on feeding practices according IYCF and IMNCI guidelines. As feeding practices differ in children of different age groups, the study population was categorized into two groups 1) 6 to 23 months of age 2) 2 to 5 years of age.

Information on indicators such as exclusive breast feeding, continued breast feeding, age at introduction of solid and semisolid food was obtained for all the children. Information on other IYCF indicators such as minimum meal frequency, minimum dietary diversity, and minimum acceptable diet was obtained for children aged between 6 to 23 months. For children between 2 to 5 years, information on feeding as per IMNCI guidelines (IMNCI 2009) was obtained. Anthropometric measurements such as height, weight and mid upper arm circumference were measured for all the children. Three standard indices of physical growth such as Weight- for-age (underweight), Height-for-age (stunting), Weight-for-height (wasting) expressed in terms of WHO Z scores were used to describe the nutritional status of children.

RESULTS

Among the study population, 47% were male and 53% were female children. The total number of children in 6 to 23 months were 66, and 2 to 5 years were 115. Among all, majority (88.4%) received exclusive breast feeding, 11.6% children received artificial feeding along with breast milk in the first 6 months of age (table 1). In 74 % of the children, introduction of solid and semisolid feeding was in the 6th month of their age. In 26% of children it was delayed beyond 6 months. Table no 2 shows that 80 % of the children had 4 or more (out of seven) types of food groups included in their diet as per the definition of the Minimum diversity of foods by WHO under IYCF guidelines however only 19.7% of children were consuming less than 4 varieties of food groups in their diet. Regarding the meal frequency, 71.2 % children were consuming meals more than required minimum number or frequency. Only 48.5% of children were taking at least or more than minimum acceptable diet. Table no.3 shows that 62.6% of the children in the age group of 2 yrs to 5 yrs were taking 3 meals and 2 nutritious foods per day as per IMNCI guidelines. Majority of them (86.2%) were taking feeds on their own, 13.8% were being fed by parents or care taker. Sharing of food from the same plate along with other children or parents was observed in 9.2%.

Anthropometric Measurements

Figure no.1 shows the height and weight distribution of the study population. Mean weight of study children was at -1.99 Z score and mean height was at -2.17 Z score.

Table 1. Breast feeding and complimentary feeding practices of tribal children

Breast feeding	Number (%) n=181
Exclusive breast feed	160(88.4)
Artificial feed along with breast	21(11.6)
Continued breast feeding	Number (%) n=181
<1yr	34(18.7)
1-2yrs	37(20.5)
>2yrs	110(60.8)
Age at Initiation of solid or semisolid feeds	Number (%) n=181
5 months	7 (3.9)
6 months	134 (74)
7 months	27 (14.9)
8 months	8 (4.4)
9 months	3 (1.7)
12 months	2 (1.1)

Table 2. IYCF indicators in children between 6 to 24 months of age

Minimum dietary diversity	Number (%) n=66
Taking diet with more than Minimum dietary diversity	53 (80.3)
Not taking diet with Minimum dietary diversity	13 (19.7)
Minimum meal frequency	Number (%) n=66
Taking diet with more than Minimum meal frequency	47 (71.2)
Not taking diet with minimum meal frequency	19 (28.8)
Minimum acceptable diet	Number (%) n=66
Taking diet with more than minimum acceptable diet	32 (48.5)
Not taking diet with minimum acceptable diet	34 (51.5)

Table 3. Feeding practices of children above 2yrs - 5yrs of age

Frequency of intake of meals	Number (%) n=115
Taking 3 meals and 2 nutritious foods per day	72 (62.6)
Not taking 3 meals and 2 nutritious foods per day	43 (37.4)
Feeding practice	Number (%) n=115
Self-feeding	99 (86.2)
feeding by care taker	16 (13.8)
Shared feeding in same plate	Number (%) n=115
Yes	11 (9.2)
No	104 (90.8)

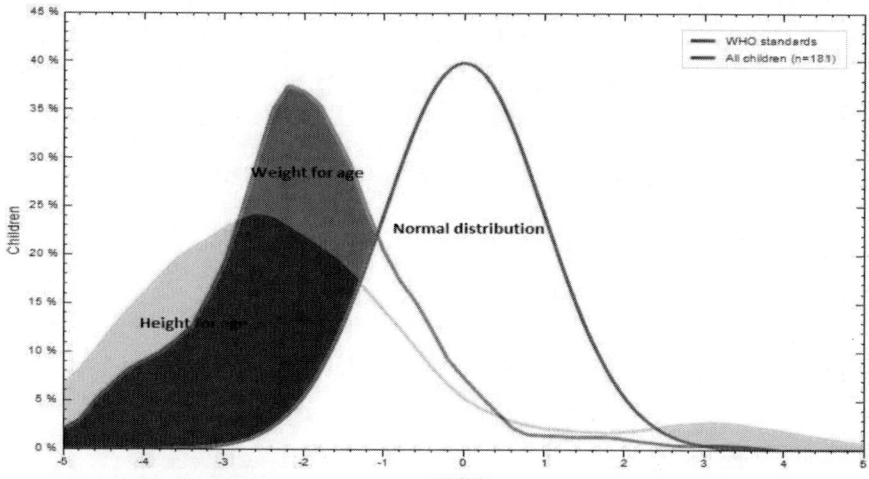

Figure 1. Distribution of Height and Weight of Study children.

Table no. 4 shows that almost half of the children (49.2%) were underweight i.e., weight for age less than < - 2 of WHO Z score. Among the underweight, 32.5% were severely underweight. Except for the first 12 months, in all other age groups around half of the study children had weight for age below -2 of WHO Z score.

The prevalence of underweight was high in 13-24 and 25-36 months of age (59% & 55.1% respectively). As shown in the above table no 5, 59% of the study children were stunted i.e., they had height for age < -2 of WHO Z score.

Among them, 64.5% had severe stunting (< -3of WHO Z score), which was more observed in 49 - 60 months age group.

Regarding weight for height, table no. 6 shows that 22.2% the study children had wasting i.e., their weight for height less than < -2 of WHO Z score.

Among them, 35% had severe wasting (<-3of WHO Z score). Wasting was more prevalent in 13 - 24 months of age. Out of 181 children 100 children (55.24%) were with MUAC < 13.5cm.

Table 4. Prevalence of Underweight in study children

Age groups	Total number of children	Normal n (%)	Under weight < -2 of WHO Z score n (%)	Severe Underweight among underweight
6-12 months	33	22 (66.7)	11(33.3)	5 (45.45)
13-24 months	39	16 (41)	23 (59)	7(30.43)
25-36 months	49	22 (44.9)	27 (55.1)	11(40.7)
37-48 months	29	15 (51.7)	14 (48.3)	1 (7.14)
49-60 months	31	17 (54.8)	14 (45.2)	5 (35.71)
Total	181	92 (50.8)	89 (49.2)	29 (32.58)

Table 5. Prevalence of stunting in study children

Age groups	Total number of children	Normal n (%)	Stunting <-2 of WHO Z score n %)	Severe stunting among stunting < -3 of WHO Z score n (%)
6-12 months	33	21(62.5)	12(37.5)	7(58.33)
13-24 months	39	23 (59)	16 (41.0)	11 (68.75)
25-36 months	49	18 (38.3)	31 (61.7)	24 (77.41)
37-48 months	29	9 (31)	20 (69.0)	7(35)
49-60 months	31	3 (9.7)	28 (90.3)	21 (75)
Total	181	74 (41)	107 (59.0)	69 (64.48)

Table 6. Prevalence of wasting in study children

Age groups	Total number of Children	Normal n (%)	Wasting <-2 of WHO Z score n (%)	Severe wasting among wasting < -3 of WHO Z score n (%)
6-12 months	33	25 (75.9)	8 (24.1)	2 (25)
13-24 months	39	19 (48.7)	20 (51.3)	11 (55)
25-36 months	49	41 (83.7)	8 (16.3)	1 (12.5)
37-48 months	29	25 (86.2)	4 (13.8)	0 (0)
49-60 months	31	0 (0)	0 (0)	0 (0)
Total	181	141(77.8)	40(22.2)	14(3.5)

Discussion

Feeding Practices of Tribal Children

It was observed that during the first six months of age of the study children, majority (88.4%) received exclusive breast milk. Among the tribal people, the practice of consuming cow or buffalo milk or any other dairy product is very negligible. Even for the purpose of feeding infants and young children mothers depend on breast milk as compared to other sources indicating a positive cultural factor benefitting the health of the new born. However this finding is in contrast to other studies which reported a poor percentage of exclusive breast feeding among other tribes. It was reported as low as 20.8% among Kol tribes of Madhya Pradesh by Tiwari et al. (2007) where as in studies by Burhanuddin et al. (2011), Mondal et al. (2014) and Sinhababu et al. (2010) it was between 31 % to 57%. The child rearing practices followed by the tribal women in our study are favorable to the children. Practice of introduction of solid or semisolid food (complimentary foods) by six months of age was observed in 74 % of children. This is similar to finding of Laxmiah et al. (2007) who reported it as 76%. Other studies among Santals by Mondal et al. (2014) and among tribes of Bankura district by Sinha babu et al. (2010) reported it as 46.6%and 55.7% respectively.

Regarding the IYCF practices, most of the children in the age group of 6 – 24 months received more than 4 types of food groups such as grains, roots, legumes, fruits, dairy products, eggs and flesh food in their diet. Mothers of more than 80% of the children demonstrated Minimum dietary diversity. Also majority of the children were receiving foods more than the recommended number of times in a day for their age. In contrast to this finding, Mondal et al. (2014) has reported a low minimum dietary diversity standards (30.85%) and minimum meal frequency (41.49%) in their study. However in the present study it is observed that only half (48.5%) of the children had minimum acceptable diet ie having both minimum dietary diversity and minimum meal frequency. Which means rest of the children were either receiving more food groups less frequently in a day or less food groups more number of times in a day. Therefore mothers need to be educated on these IYCF guidelines (WHO 2008) to include more food groups and feed as frequently as advised.

Regarding feeding practices of children more than 24 months, IMNCI recommends at least 3 meals and 2 nutritious foods per day. In this study 62.6% of the children of 2 years to 5 years, were receiving adequate frequent meals as per the IMNCI guidelines (2009) and 90.8 % were had separate plate for food. Majority of them (86.2%) were taking feeds on their own.

Nutritional Status of Tribal Children

In our study, the prevalence of underweight among children under five was found to be 49.2%. Among the underweight, 35.29% were severely underweight (< -3 of WHO Z score). The age wise weight distribution of the children shows that less percentage of children were underweight during their infancy and as the age progresses more number of children are falling in to the bracket of underweight. This can be attributed to the fact that practices such exclusive breast feeding and timely initiation of complimentary feeds are keeping the infant well-nourished but as age progresses and the milk feed is slowly withdrawn, the quantity of food supplementation are not adequate to meet the demands of the young child's growth and development thus forcing him into the bracket of underweight. Other studies (Sinhababu et al. 2010) have also attributed the problem of underweight to inappropriate complementary feeding practices along with late initiation and low rates of breast feeding.

Height for age index reflects chronic energy deficiency. In this study, it is observed that the percentage of children being stunted increases as the age progresses which means children in the younger age groups being well nourished are gaining good height but as the age progresses, due to inadequate complimentary feeds; they gradually end up having low height for their age or severe stunting.

However the weight for height index (wasting) indicating acute malnutrition shows that more percentage of children in the 13 – 24 months is wasted.

This is the critical age bracket where the inadequacy in the complimentary feeds directly affects the weight of the child leading to acute malnutrition. Gradually it is found to be zero in the older age groups suggesting that for the low height gained over a period of time, weight for that height is normal. According to Mid upper arm circumference, out of 181 children 100 children (55.24%) were malnourished i.e., were having < 13.5cm.

CONCLUSION

Tribals follow child friendly feeding practices as reflected in the breast feeding and weaning practices. It is understood from this study that feeding practices in the early infancy are satisfactory. However as the child grows old, there is deficiency in the frequency and adequacy of the feeds because of which the child becomes wasted and stunted. Reasons for which may be poverty, illiteracy and non-accessibility to nutritious foods and health education.

ACKNOWLEDGMENTS

I am especially thankful to Addl DM&HO of ITDA Paderu for giving his support and we are also thankful to the Medical Officers of selected PHCs for providing health care staff to conduct the study.

REFERENCES

Burhanuddin, M., Rahman, S. M. B., Imtiaz Hussain. Infants Feeding Practices among Garo and non Garo Mothers from Netrakona District Bangladesh. *World Journal of Medical Sciences*, 2011; 6(4); 202 - 208.

Integrated management of neonatal and childhood illness (imnci) Modules 1 to 9. New delhi. *Ministry of health and family welfare.* Government of india. 2009. P. 356.

Laxmaiah, A., Mallikharjuna, Rao K., Hari Kumar, R., Arlappa, N., Venkaiah, K., G. N. V. Brahmam. Diet and Nutritional Status of Tribal Population in ITDA Project Areas of Khammam District, Andhra Pradesh. *J. Hum. Ecol.,* 2007 21(2): 79 - 86.

Ministry of Tribal Affairs. *Demographic Status of Scheduled Tribe Population of India* [*internet*]. Available from: http://tribal.nic.in/Write ReadData/CMS/Documents/201306110208002203443DemographicSta tusofScheduledTribeP opulationofIndia.pdf.

Ministry of Women and Child development. *Scheduled Tribe Women and Children: Issues and challenges for development.* New Delhi; Ministry of Women and Child development. 2011. Available from: http://www.p ib.nic.in/newsite/erelease.aspx?relid=72382.

Mondal, T. K., Sarkar, A. P., Shivam, S., Thakur, R. P. Assessment of infant and young child feeding practice among tribal women in Bhatkar block of Burdwan district in West Bengal, India. *Int. J. Med. Sci. Public Health,* 2014; 3; 324 - 326.

Sinhababu, A., Dipta, K. Mukhopadhyay, Tanmay K. Panja, Asit B. Saren, Nirmal K. Mandal, Akhil B. Biswas. Infant and Young Child-feeding

Practices in Bankura District, West Bengal, India. *J. Health popul. Nutr.*, 2010 Jun.; 28(3):294 - 299.

Tiwari, B. K., Rao, V. G., Mishra, D. K., Thakur, C. Infant-feeding practices among Kol tribal community of Madhya Pradesh. *Indian J. Community Med.,* 2007; 32:228 - 228.

Varadarajan, A., Prasad, S., Regional variations in Nutritional Status among tribals of Andhra Pradesh, *Stud Tribes Tribals,* 2009; 7(2): p. 137 - 141.

World Health Organaization. 2008. *Indicators for assessing infant and young child feeding practices part 1 Definitions*. France. Pp. 26.

In: Contemporary Issues in Childhood … ISBN: 978-1-53617-348-2
Editors: J. Ratan Ghosh and K. Bose ©2020 Nova Science Publishers, Inc.

Chapter 10

Factors Affecting Thinness among Children of Purba Medinipur, West Bengal

Pikli Khanra[1], Kaushik Bose[1,*] and Jyoti Ratan Ghosh[2]
[1]Department of Anthropology, Vidyasagar University, Midnapore, West Bengal, India
[2]Department of Anthropology, Visva-Bharati University, Santiniketan, West Bengal India

Abstract

The present study was conducted to understand the prevalence of thinness and its associations with socio-economic and demographic characteristics among school children. A total of 552 boys and 567 girls aged between 3 and 11 years from Haldia and Deshopran of Purba Medinipur districe, West Bengal were incorporated in the present cross-sectional study. The overall prevalence of thinness was 67.74%. However, the prevalence of thinness was lower among boys (66.12%) compared to girls (69.31%). Binary logistic regression analysis revealed that parents

*Corresponding Author's Email: kaushikbose@cantab.net.

education, fathers occupation, sanitation, number of living room and illness were significantly ($p < 0.05$) associated with thinness.

Step-wise logistic regression analysis demonstrated that father occupation, illness and sanitation were also significantly ($p < 0.05$) associated with thinness.

Keywords: children, BMI, thinness, socio-economic and demographic factors

INTRODUCTION

Undernutrition is the leading cause of morbidity and mortality in infants, children and adolescents throughout the world (Demissie and Work 2013, Meshram et al., 2012, Global Nutrition Report 2018). It has been estimated that approximately two-thirds of the world's undernourished children live in Asia with highest concentration of worldwide childhood undernutrition (Ramachandran 2014; UNICEF 2016). Undernutrition continues to cause nearly half of deaths in children aged less than 5 years, which have a significant effect on human health as well as social, economic and political development (Black et al., 2003, Global Nutrition Report 2016). The health consequences of a prolonged state of undernutrition among children include delayed physical growth, impaired intellect, lower resistances to infection and high risk for some chronic diseases, which also hampered work capacity, reproductive performance and behavioral status (Park 2007, Masibo and Makoka 2012, Mengistu et al., 2013, Singh et al., 2013). Undernutrition is also associated with diseases like measles, diarrhea and acute respiratory infectious disease (Meshram et al., 2012, Demissie and Work 2013).

Undernutrition explains around 45% of deaths among children under five, mainly in low and middle-income countries (Global Nutrition Report 2018). Undenutrution is also a major problem challenging India. In India, there are about 60 million underweight children and its prevalence is higher in rural areas compared to the urban areas (Smith et al., 2005, Herrador et al., 2014). However, a number of programs have been launched to control the situation, such as ICDS (launched in 1974) and "Mid-day meal Program" to improv children and maternal health status. It was observed that thinness was a comparatively better indicator than wasting among children to assess the undernourition (Cole et al., 2007) and the chronic energy deficiency (CED), grades III, II and I of thinness, refer to severe, moderate and mild under nutrition, respectively. Undernutrition among school children is an important public health problem of any country (Rana et al. 2012, Mansur et al., 2014, Teblick et al., 2017). However, information on thinness among children of developing countries like in India is important because a large number of people in India are suffering from undrenutrition. Several studies have reported that the prevalence of thinness was high in India (Singh and Mondal 2013, Singh et al., 2014, Vaidya et al., 2015, Selvaraj et al., 2016, Bharati et al., 2017). Higher prevalence of thinness was also observed among children of West Bengal (Mondal et al., 2009, Banik and Chatterjee 2010, Mandal et al., 2014, Giri et al., 2017).

The prevalence of thinness may influence by a number of factors including access to water, sanitation and hygiene, income, education and quality health services (Yadav et al., 2016, Pal et al., 2016, Pal et al., 2017, Gurzkowska et al., 2017, Global Nutrition 2016-2017 and Child Mortality, 2017; Debnath et al., 2018, Global Nutrition Report 2018). However, little information is available on the nutritional status of children in West Bengal. Therefore, the aim of the present study was to understand the prevalence of undernutrition and its association with socio-economic and demographic characteristics among school children.

MATERIALS AND METHODS

The present cross-sectional study was conducted in Haldia and Deshopran of Purba Medinipur and the data was collected during the period December 2014 to April 2016. The study was conducted in 1119 children aged 3-11 years and selected through door to door visits. Out of the total participants 552 (49.33%) were boys and 567 (50.67%) were girls.

Height and weight of the participants were measured by standard techniques (Lohman et al., 1988). Height was measured to the nearest of

0.10 cm by using an anthropometer and weight was measured to the nearest 0.50 kg by using a weighing machine. BMI (Body mass index) was calculated from the height and weight using following equation- BMI (kg/m^2) = weight/(kg)/height $(m)^2$. Nutritional status was evaluated using anthropometric indicators recommended by Cole et al. (2007). Nutritional status was evaluated using the age and sex specific cut-off points of BMI for children (Cole et al., 2007). The chronic energy deficiency (CED) grade III, II and I of thinness refer to severe, moderate and mild under nutrition, respectively. Socio demographic and socio-economic variables including family size (number of family member), earning members, living room, illness, parental education, parental occupation, income and expenditure were collected by using a pre-structured questioner.

The numerical data were presented as mean ± SD. Student's t test was used to compare the means. One-way analysis of variance (ANOVA) was done to assess difference between mean values of anthropometric measurements within age groups. Chi-squre test was used to assess sex difference in the prevalence of nutritional status. Binary logistic regression (BLR, i.e., univariate analysis) was used to determine the relationship between thinness with socio-economic and socio-demographic factors and to estimate odd ratios (ORs). The predictor variables entered in the regression equation includes parental education (above secondary and up to secondary), father occupation (manual and non-manual), mother occupation (non-manual, house wife, manual), house ownership (own and rental), number of living room (>2 rooms, ≤2 rooms), family size (≤5 members, >5 members), earning members (≥4 members, 2-3 members, 1members), sanitation (properly present, not properly present), illness (above five month and within five month), per capita monthly family income (≤Rs. 1750, >Rs. 1750) and monthly family expenditure per capita (≤Rs. 2000, >Rs. 2000). All statistical analyses were done using SPSS version 16.

Table 1. Mean and stander deviation of weight, height and BMI among participant

Age (Years)	Boys				Girls			
	n	Mean Weight [kg] (SD)	Mean Height [cm] (SD)	Mean BMI [kg/m²] (SD)	n	Mean Weight [kg] (SD)	Mean Height [cm] (SD)	Mean BMI [kg/m²] (SD)
3	61	13.00 (1.82)	99.75 (5.37)	13.05 (1.42)	61	13.04 (2.04)	100.82 (7.21)	12.78 (1.61)
4	62	13.92 (2.48)	101.70 (6.42)	13.38 (1.47)	61	14.26 (2.38)	104.22 (7.45)	13.10 (1.45)
5	60	16.09 (2.75)	109.43 (5.91)	13.39 (1.53)	66	15.37 (2.50)	108.17 (6.24)	13.09 (1.46)
6	63	17.58 (2.78)	113.44 (5.06)	13.63 (1.66)	62	17.05 (2.97)	112.34 (4.92)	13.52 (2.22)
7	61	18.47 (3.02)	115.94 (5.69)	13.69 (1.46)	61	18.12 (3.54)	115.19 (6.13)	13.57 (1.80)
8	61	20.69 (3.07)	122.22 (6.84)	13.82 (1.43)	63	20.23 (3.91)	120.84 (7.71)	13.77 (1.69)
9	60	23.80 (4.43)	126.99 (8.21)	14.68 (1.74)	62	21.72 (4.63)	123.52 (8.49)	14.08 (1.52)
10	61	25.50 (5.48)	131.37 (8.72)	14.65 (1.99)	68	25.28 (6.29)	129.96 (8.82)	14.77 (2.27)
11	63	29.25 (7.15)	136.72 (9.37)	15.44 (2.28)	63	28.14 (6.19)	135.39 (9.55)	15.15 (1.79)
ANOVA		114.96^{***}	207.86^{***}	13.19^{***}		94.75^{***}	151.79^{***}	12.43^{***}

n = No. of Participant; SD = Standard deviation; ANOVA p^{***} = <0.001.

RESULTS

Mean and stander deviation of anthropometric characteristics of the studied population are presented in Table 1. Results of ANOVA showed that mean values of height, weight and BMI were significantly ($p < 0.001$) varried according to age groups. Student's t-test demonstrated (Table 2) that girls were significantly taller than boys at the age of 4 years ($p < 0.05$). Contrary to that, at 9 years boys were significantly taller and heavier than girls ($p < 0.05$).

Table 2. Sex difference between mean value of weight, height and BMI

Age (Years)	P values for difference in mean weight, height & BMI of boys & girls		
	t	t	t
3	-0.10	-0.93	0.97
4	-0.77	-2.01*	1.06
5	1.54	1.16	1.11
6	1.04	1.23	0.29
7	0.59	0.70	0.38
8	0.74	1.06	0.19
9	2.54**	2.30*	2.02*
10	0.21	0.91	-0.29
11	0.93	0.79	0.77

$p^{*} = <0.05$, $p^{**} < 0.01$.

Table 3. Prevalence of thinness among studied children using BMI

Categories	Boys (n = 552)	Girls (n = 567)	Total (n = 1119)	df	X^2
Grade-I	140 (25.36)	153 (26.98)	293 (26.18)	1	0.58
Grade-II	73 (13.22)	94 (16.58)	167 (14.92)	1	2.64
Grade-III	152 (27.54)	146 (25.75)	298 (26.63)	1	0.12
Overall Thinness	365 (66.12)	393 (69.31)	758 (67.74)	1	1.03
Normal	187 (33.88)	174 (30.69)	361 (32.26)	1	0.47

n = No. of participant; df = Degree of freedom.

Table 3 shows that 67.74% children were thin and 32.26% children were normal. Higher prevalence of Grade-I and Grade-II thinness was observed in girls compared to boys, however the prevalence of Grade-III thinness was higher in boys compared to girls. However, the overall prevalence of thinness was higher in girls compared to boys.

The results of the BLR analysis demonstrated greater odds ratio for number of earning member, income, expenditure and mother occupation for being thin ($p > 0.05$). Children, who suffered from diseases within 5 months demonstrated 1.42 times greater risk ($p < 0.01$) for thinness.However, children living in rental house demonstrated lower risk (OR = 0.71, $p < 0.05$) for thinness. Children without proper sanitation had 1.65 times ($p < 0.01$) greater risk for thinness. The odds values were also significantly higher (1.49 times, $p < 0.01$) for thinness among children with ≤2 living rooms. The larger family size had a lower risk OR = 0.97, $p > 0.05$) for thinness. The odds of thinness were also significantly greater among children whose fathers were manual worker (1.46 times, $p < 0.01$) and had up to secondary parental education (mother, OR = 1.43, $p < 0.05$; father, OR = 1.45, $p < 0.01$). The result of step-wise logistic regression analyses (forward conditional model) to determine the independent socio-economic and demographic factors for thinness (Table 5) showed significantly ($p < 0.01$) higher odds for whose fathers were laboure. Similarly children who were ill within five months also had higher ($p < 0.01$) risk for thinness. Children without proper sanitary system (odds 1.46, $p < 0.05$) also had higher risk for thinness.

DISCUSSION

India has great opportunity to improve the health and nutritional status of its citizens because of the economic development that occurred in the last two or three decades. Though, there were impressive improvements in India in terms of reduction in fertility rate and infant mortality rate, improvement in health and nutritional status were not satisfactory. Several programs have been lunched for the improvement of child health and nutrition in India. But, more than half of undernourished population of the world lives in India (Krishnaswami 2000). Inequitable distribution of poverty, demographic and socio-economic condition reflects on health. Undernutrition is an indicator of poor nutrition and health of any population. Previous studies on undernutrition among children in West Bengal showed that a large number of children were suffering form undernutrition.

In the present study, overall prevalence of thinness was 67.74% based on Cole reference values. However, the overall prevalence of thinness among participants was very high compared to the children of Bangladesh (30.88%), Tanzania (11.30%), Nigeria (9.29%) and Nepal (10.50%). High prevalence of thinness was also observed in the present study compared to studies of Singh and Mondal 2013, (25.99%), Singh et al., 2014 (36.18%),

Vaidya et al., 2015 (32.10%), Eze et al., 2017 (9.29%), Das et al., 2009 (48.40%), Banik et al., 2010 (23.84%) and Selvaraj et al., 2016 (17.90%).

Table 4. Binary logistic regression analysis, demographic, socio-economic and life style factors affecting on thinness

Variables	Categories	n	Thinness	(%)	B	Wald	OR	95.0% C. I.
Family Size (No. of Family Members)	<5®	813	552	67.90	-	-	-	1
	≥5	306	206	67.32	-0.03	0.03	0.97	0.74-1.29
Expenditure	>1750 Rs®	530	354	66.79	-	-	-	1
	≤1750 Rs.	589	404	68.59	0.08	0.41	1.09	0.85-1.39
Income	>2000 Rs®	623	419	67.26	-	-	-	1
	≤2000 Rs.	496	339	68.35	0.05	0.15	1.05	0.82-1.35
Illness	Above Five Month®	423	266	62.88	-	-	-	1
	Within Five Month	696	492	70.69	0.35	7.31	1.42**	1.10-1.84
House Ownership	Own®	871	605	69.46	-	-	-	1
	Rental	248	153	61.69	-0.35	5.3	0.71*	0.53-0.95
Sanitation	Properly Present®	922	608	65.94	-	-	-	1
	Not Properly Present	197	150	76.14	0.50	7.62	1.65**	1.16-2.35
No. of living Rooms	>2®	231	140	60.61	-	-	-	1
	≤2	888	618	69.59	0.39	6.73	1.49**	1.10-2.00
Earning Members	>1®	284	189	66.55	-	-	-	1
	1	835	569	68.14	0.07	0.20	1.07	0.16-1.51
Mother Occupation	Non-Manual®	112	73	65.18	-	-	-	1
	House Wife	973	657	67.52	0.11	0.25	1.11	0.74-1.68
	Manual	34	28	82.35	0.91	3.45	2.49	0.95-6.54
Father Occupation	Non-Manual®	481	303	62.99	-	-	-	1
	Manual	638	455	71.32	0.38	8.66	1.46**	1.14-1.88
Mother Education	Above Secondary®	230	141	61.30	-	-	-	1
	Up to Secondary	889	617	69.40	0.36	5.45	1.43*	1.06-1.94
Father Education	Above Secondary®	322	199	61.80	-	-	-	1
	Up to Secondary	797	559	70.14	0.37	7.26	1.45**	1.11-1.90

n = No. of participant, (%) = Values in parentheses; OR = Odds ratio; C. I. = Confidence intervals.

Table 5. Factors associated with thinness among school going children

Variables	Categories	OR (95%CI) (Step-1)	OR (95%CI) (Step-2)	OR (95%) (Step-3)
Father Occupation	Non-Manual®	-	-	-
	Manual	1.46** (1.14-1.88)	1.47** (1.14-1.89)	1.40** (1.08-1.81)
Illness	Above Five Month®		-	-
	Within Five Month		1.44** (1.11-1.86)	1.39** (1.08-1.81)
Sanitation	Properly Present®			-
	Not Properly Present			1.46* (1.01-2.09)

OR = Odds ratio; CI = Confidence intervals.

Another study among children of Karnataka revealed that 61.7% children were thin (Nayak et al., 2015) and this prevalence was lower than the present study. The study by Mondal et al., (2009) reported 85.16% children were nutritionally thin as well as another recent study in children of Sagar block revealed 81.25% (Giri et al., 2017) children were thin, all these prevalence were very high than the present study.

There are numerous and multifaceted causes of thinness and these causes are interrelated with each other. In the present study, larger family size (≥5 individuals) had lower risks for thinness ($p < 0.05$). But some previous studies reported that large family size had a greater risk for thinness (Mondal and Sen 2010, Mondal et al., 2015, Yadav et al., 2016, Pal et al., 2017). In the present study, the odds for thinness were found greater among children belonging to low monthly family income. Similar studies also reported that the children belonging to lower income households were found to be a greater risk for thinness (Mondal and Sen 2010, Mondal et al., 2015, Yadav et al., 2016, Pal et al., 2017). In the present study low monthly per capita expenditure had greater odds (1.09 times) for thinness. Those children who were ill within five months also had significantly ($p < 0.01$) higher risk (1.42 times) for thinness. The significantly ($p < 0.01$) greater odds (1.65 times) for thinness was found in children those had no proper sanitation facility. Similarly, some studies had reported that sanitation (not properly present) had greater risk for thinness (Yadav et al., 2016, Pal et al., 2016, Pal et al., 2017). In the present study the odds for thinness was significantly greater (1.49 times, $p < 0.01$) among children having lower ($\leq$2 room) categories of living room. Few previous studies had reported an association between living room and greater risk for thinness (Debnath et al., 2018). The greater risk of parental occupation on the prevalence of thinness was also observed in the present study. The children whose parents were labour had higher risk for thinness. Some previous studies also reported that significant association of parental occupation and child nutrition (Mondal et al., 2015, Pal et al., 2016, Selvaraj et al., 2016, Pal et al., 2017, Debnath et al., 2018). Significantly greater (1.42 and 1.45 times) effect of parental education on child nutrition was also found in the present study. Similarly, some previous studies also observed that parental education was significantly associated with child malnutrition (Meshram et al., 2012, Pal et al., 2016, Selvaraj et al., 2016, Yadav et al., 2016, Pal et al., 2017, Tariku et al., 2018).

Conclusion

India has many challenges in improving the health of its citizens. Many aspects, such as the fertility rate, maternal mortality and infant and child mortality rate are declining. The present study showed that 67.74% children were nutritionally thin and also showed that socially, economically and educationally weaker sections of the population were more likely to be thin. Thus, immideat nutritional intervention is necessary to improve the nutritional status among the children.

Recommendations

The present study recommends for urgent iniatives for awareness programme on health and child nutrition both in rural and urban areas. However, it is only possible when government, non-governmental organizations, medical persons and health workers along with local people will work together to manage it.

LIMITATIONS

The present study had some limitations including its cross-sectional nature as well as unavailability of data on mother health condition of the participants, parasitic infection, and type of food consumption, and physical activity which may have an important effect on childhood malnutrition.

ACKNOWLEDGMENTS

The authors are greatfulto B. D. O. of Desopran block and Chairperson of Haldia Municipality for given permission to conduct the study. Authors are also greatful to all the participants.

REFERENCES

Alazzeh AY, AlShammari EM, Smadi MM, Azzch FS, AlShammari BT, Epuru S, Banu S, Bano R, Sulaiman S, Alcantara JC, Ashraf SA and Qiblawi S. 2018. Some Socio-economic Factors and Lifestyle Habits Influencing the Prevalence of Obesity among Adolescent Male Students in the Hail Region of Saudi Arabia.*Children*. 39(5):1-10.

Banik SD, Chatterjee S. 2010. Nutritional status of school going children and adolescents aged 9-13 years at Haldia in West Bengal, India. *Paediatr. Indones.*, 50 (3):159-165.

Bann D, Johnson W, Li L, Kuh D, Hardy R. 2018. Socio-economic inequalities in childhood and adolescent body-mass index, weight, and height from 1953 to 2015: an analysis of four longitudinal, observational, British birth cohort studies. *Lancet.* 3: e194-203.

Bharthi K, Ghritlahre M, Das S, Bose K. 2017. Nutritional status among children and adolescents aged 6-18 years of Kolam tribe of Andhra Pradesh, India. *Anthropol. Rev*. 80(2): 153-163.

Black RE, Morris SS, Bryce J. 2003. Where and why are 10 million children dying every year? *Lancet*. 351:2226-34.

Child Mortality Report. 2017. *Levels & Trends in Estimates Developed by the UN Inter-agency Group for Child Mortality Estimation*. New York.

Cole TJ, Flegal KM, Nicholls D, Jackson AA. 2007. Body mass index cut offs to define thinness in children and adolescents: international survey. *BMJ*. 335: 194.

Das S and K Bose. 2009. Anthropometric Characteristics and Nutritional Status of Bauri Pre-School Children of Nituria Block, Purulia, West Bengal. *Internet. J. Biol. Anthropol.* 3(2):16-6.

Debnath S, Mondal N and Sen J. 2018. Socio-economic and Demographic Correlates of Stunting and Thinness among Rural School-going Children (Aged 5-12 Years) of North Bengal, Eastern India. *J. Life Science*. 10(1): 29-46.

Degarege D, Degarege A, Animut A. 2015. Undernutrition and associated risk factors among school age children in Addis Ababa, Ethiopia.*BMC Public Health*.15:375.

Demissie S, Work A. 2013. Magnitude and Factors Associated with Malnutrition in Children 6-59 Months of Age in Pastoral Community of Dollo Ado District, Somali Region, Ethiopia. *Sci. J. Public Health*. 1:175-183.

Eze JN, Oguonu T, Ojinnaka NC, Ibe BC. 2017. Physical growth and nutritional status assessment of school children in Enugu, Nigeria. *Niger. J. Clin. Pract*.20 (1):64-70.

Giri SP, Biswas S, Bose K. 2017. Very high prevalence of thinness among rural bengalee preschool children of integrated child development service (ICDS) scheme of Sagar Island, South 24 Parganas, West Bengal, India. *Anthropol. Open J*. 2(2):54-60.

Global Nutrition Report 2018. *Shining a light to spur action on nutrition Executive Summary*. Yangambi, Democratic Republic of the Congo.

Girls carrying vegetables. International Forestry Research. Bristol, UK: Development Initiatives.

Global Nutrition Report 2016. *From To Promise Impact Ending Malnutrition By 2030.* A peer-reviewed publication. International Food Policy Research Institute. Washington.

Grebmer K. V., Bernstein J., Patterson F., Sonntag A., Klaus L. M., Fahlbusch J., Towey O. 2018. *The concept of the Global hunger index. Laura Hammond,* SOAS University of London Dublin.

Gurzkowska B, Kułaga Z, Grajda A, GozdzWojtyłoM, Litwin M. 2017. The relationship between selected socioeconomic factors and thinness among Polish school-aged children and adolescents. *Eur. J. Pediatr.* 176:797-806.

Herrador Z, Sordo L, Gadisa E, Moreno J, Nieto J, Benito A, et al. 2014. Cross-Sectional study of malnutrition and associated factors among school aged children in rural and urban settings of Fogera and LiboKemkem Districts, Ethiopia. *PloS One.* 9(9):e105880.

Krishnaswami K. 2000. Country profile; India nutritional disorders old and changing. *Lancet* 315:1268-9.

Makoka D, 2013. *The Impact of Maternal Education on Child Nutrition:* Evidence from Malawi, Tanzania, and Zimbabwe ICF International Calverton, Maryland, USA, University of Malawi.

Mansur DI, Haque MK, Sharma K, Mehta DK, Shakya R. 2015. A Study on Nutritional Status of Rural School going Children in Kavre District.*Kathmandu Univ. Med. J.* 50(2):146-151.

Mandal GC, Bose K and Bisai S. 2009. Thinness among Rural Children in Bengal. *Ind. J. Pediatr.* 76 (8): 817-819.

Mandal S, Prabhakar VR, Pal J, Parthasarathi R, Biswas R. 2014. An assessment of nutritional status of children aged 0-14 years in a slum area of Kolkata. *Int. J. Med. and Public Health.* 4 (2):159-162.

Masibo PK, Makoka D. 2012. Trends and determinants of undernutrition among young Kenyan children: Kenya Demographic and Health Survey: 1993, 1998, 2003 and 2008-2009. *Public Health Nutr.* 15:1715-1727.

Melaku YA, Zello GA, Gill TK, Adams RJ, Shi Z. 2015. Prevalence and factors associated with stunting and thinness among adolescent students in Northern Ethopia: a comparison to World Health Organization standards. *Arch. Public Health*. 73-44.

Mengistu K, Alemu K, Destaw B. 2013. Prevalence of malnutrition and associated factors among children aged 6-59 Months at HidabuAbote district, North Shewa, Oromia regional state. *J. Nutr. Disord. Ther.* T1:001.

Meshram II, Arlappa N, Balakrishna N Rao KM, Laxmaiah A, Brahman GNV. 2012. Trends in the prevalence of undernutrition, nutrient and food intake and predictors of undernutrition among under five year tribal children in India. *Asia Pac. J. Clin. Nutr*. 21:568-576.

Mitra M, Kumar PV, Chakrabarty S, Bharati P. 2007. Nutritional status of kamar tribal children in Chhatisgarh. *Ind. J. Pediatr*. 74:381-384.

Mondal N, Sen J. 2010. Prevalence of stunting and thinness among rural adolescents of Darjeeling district, West Bengal, India. *Ital. J. Pub. Health*. 7: 54-61.

Mondal N, Sen J. 2010. Prevalence of under-nutrition among children (5-12 years) belonging to three communities residing in a similar habitat in North Bengal, India. *Ann. Hum. Biol*. 37: 199-217.

Mondal N, Basumatary B, Kropi J, Bose K. 2015. Prevalence of double burden of malnutrition among urban school going Bodo children aged 5-11 years of Assam, Northeast India. *Epidemiology Biostatistics and Public Health*. 12:e11497-1-10.

National Family Health Survey (NFHS-4), 2015-16, National Report, International Institute of population Science, Mumbai, India.

Nayak RK, Walvekar PR, Mallapur MD. 2015. Thinness among preschool children residingin rural area: A cross-sectional study. *J. Scientific Society*. 42 (2):78-81.

Pal D, Kanugo S, Bal B, Bhowmik K, Mahapatra T and Sarkar K. 2016. Malnutrition seenario among school children in Eastern-India-an Epidemiological study. *Epidemiology (Sunnyvale)*.6(2):1-9.

Pal A, Pari AK, Sinha A, Dhara PC. Prevalence of undernutrition and associated factors: A cross-sectional study among rural adolescents in

West Bengal, India. *Int. J. Pediatrics and Adolescent Med.* 2017; 4:9-18.

Park K. 2005. Park's textbook of preventive and social medicine, 18thed., Jabalpur; Banarasidas Bhanot Publishers. P. 405.

Pramanik P, Banerjee SB, Dey S. 2015. Prevalence of Under Nutrition and Poor Health Status among Primary School Children in Burdwan West Bengal. *Sch. J. App. Med. Sci.* 3(5A):1851-1857.

Ramachandran N 2014.Persisting Undernutrition in India: Causes, Consequences and Possible Solutions.ISBN 978-81-322-1832-6 (eBook).

Rana M. M., Ferdoushi A., Tamanna S., Sabrin F., Afroz S. S. 2012. Assessment of nutritional status of 5-10 years Garo children in Sherpur District, Bangladesh. *Int. J. Biosci.* 2 (11): 66-73.

Selvaraj V, Sangareddi S, Celmurugan L, Muniyappan U, Anitha FS. 2016. Nutritional status of adolescent school children in a semi-urban area based on anthropometry. *Int. J. Contemp. Pediatr.* 3(2):468-472.

Singh JP, Gupta SB, Shrotriya VP, Singh PN. 2013. Study of nutritional status among under five children attending out patient department at a primary care rural hospital, Bareilly (UP). *Sch. J. App. Med. Sci.* 1:769-773.

Singh J, Mondal N. 2013. Assessment of Nutritional Status: A Case of Tribal Children in Assam, Northeast India. *J. Nepal Paediatr. Soc.* 33(1):1-7.

Singh1 JP, Kariwal P, Gupta SB, Singh AK, Imtiaz D. 2014. Nutritional status and morbidity among school going children: A scenario from a rural India. *Sch. J. App. Med. Sci.* 2(1D):379-383.

Smith LC, Ruel MT, Ndiaye A. 2005. Why is child malnutrition lower in urban than in rural areas? Evidence from 36 developing countries. *World Development.* 33(8): 1285-1305.

Tariku E. Z., Abebe G. A., Melketsedik Z. A., Gutema B.T. 2018. Prevalence and factors associated withstunting and thinness among school-age children in Arba Minch Health and Demographic Surveillance Site, SouthernEthiopia. *PLoS ONE.* 13(11): e0206659.

Teblick A, Deken SD, Vanderbruggen W, Vermeersch M, Teblick S, Ruymaekers M, Andries J, Colebunders R, and Mmbando BP. 2017.

Anthropometry and Nutritional Status of Primary School Children in a Sub-urban Region in Tanzania.*Int. J. School Health*. 4(3):e46079.

UNICEF, WHO, World Bank Group 2016. *Levels and Trends in Child Malnutrition in UNICEF/WHO/World Bank Group Joint Child Malnutrition Estimates Key Findings of the 2016 Edition*. New York: UNICEF; Geneva: WHO; Washington DC: World Bank.

Vaidya V, Gaware SD, Murakar SK, Mishra A, Banerjee A. 2015. Nutritional status of rural India school children of Maharashtra. *Int. J. Health Sc.* 5(5):17-21.

Yadav A.K, Kotwal A, Vaidya R, Yadav J. 2016. Anthropometric indices and its socio-demographic determinants among primary school children of an urban school in Pune, India.*Int. J. Med. Public Health*. 6(4): 160-164.

In: Contemporary Issues in Childhood … ISBN: 978-1-53617-348-2
Editors: J. Ratan Ghosh and K. Bose

Chapter 11

HEALTH STATUS OF THE RURAL CHILDREN OF PURULIA, WEST BENGAL, INDIA

Rima Ghosh[1] and Diptendu Chatterjee[2,*]
[1]Department of Nutrition,
Vidyasagar University, West Bengal, India
[2]Department of Anthropology,
University of Calcutta, West Bengal, India

ABSTRACT

India is the second highest country after China in population and it is increasing day by day. Almost all the regions suffer from different kinds of nutritional problems. The purpose of this study was to evaluate the knowledge, attitudes and behaviours about nutrition of parents with children's health status in two different socio economic groups. A fieldwork was used to collect information on health variables of children (n=185) aged 7-12 years, from two significantly opposite socio-economic groups. Anthropometric variables were used to know the children's current health status. All anthropometric parameters showed the poor health status of the children in both economic groups, which shows the inappropriate

---

[*]Corresponding Author's Email: dip_cu@rediffmail.com.

diet. The lack of diet knowledge of the parents is the main cause behind it. The study concludes that both groups of children show nutritional deficiency or imbalance as well as a visible incorrect diet and no maintenance in their good health practice by their parents.

Keywords: children, health status, rural, West Bengal

INTRODUCTION

Good nutrition is the cornerstone for child in this growing period. Children are habituated in a certain diet pattern from this age, and their choice of food also starts to develop from this age. Young children's knowledge about healthy food may influence the formation of their eating behaviors, and parents have a major influence on the development of children's knowledge in the early years (Brug, 2008). Parent's choices are also based on religion, caste and their belonging from the particular socio-economic group (Cluss, 2013).

The nutritional status has a wide range from extreme under nutrition to over nutrition (McNab et al., 2016). The energy and essential nutrients are needed for growth, development and maturation of various tissues and organs of human body, which is related to physical activity and energy expenditure. Socio-economic status has the great impact in dealing with the health of the child (Fadare, 2019).

Body Mass Index is a commonly used method for determining the obesity and under-nutrition in both adult and children (WHO, 2005) and gives a standardized category of BMI which is widely accepted (Elizabet, 1978). There are also many anthropometric tools which can be used as good indicators of health status (WHO 2005).

In all developing countries there are two significant groups: one is below poverty and another one is affluent. These two groups show complete oppose pictures in terms of child's health as well as parent's nutritional knowledge (Nirmalan, 2014). This particular study will show two types of family income levels and nutrition knowledge effect in the health status of future generations (Keys, 2015).

The objective of the present study is to evaluate the nutritional status of children with respect to their parent's nutritional awareness income level.

MATERIALS AND METHODS

The present study is a fieldwork based cross sectional study designed using purposive volunteers of children 7-12 years old with apparently healthy appearances from Purulia, West Bengal, India. Anthropometric measurements are done to the child in school. Six schools are studied in urban and city area and these children also come from different socio-economic groups (Cameron et al., 1981). This socio economic factor is divided based on Tendulkar's survey report (Tendulkar, 2019). From these 6 schools, 104 children from a lower income group and 81 children from a higher income group participated (Nanclares et al., 2018). A structured schedule/questionnaire used to talk about their socio-economic and life-style variable is used (Nmer et al., 2014). Two groups were considered depending on income level. The first is lower socio economic group (LSEG) and the second is higher socio economic group (HSEG). Anthropometric measurements were taken including height, weight, hip circumference, waist circumference, head circumference and mid-upper arm circumference following the standard technique (Weiner and Lourie, 1981). Body mass index (BMI) was derived using standard formula (kg/m^2) and cut off was followed as WHO 2005 Stunting, wasting and MUAC were calculated with Z score and percentile (Zarnowiecki et al., 2012). Martin's anthropometric measurement tools are used for this study (Nirmalan, 2014). Standardized measurement tapes and weighing machine were used to calculate body mass index, mid upper arm circumference, waist and hip circumference (Keys, 2015). Data were computed and checked. All these variables are analyzed by using necessary statistics and software (Zarnowiecki et al., 2012).

Table 1. Distribution of height according to age

Age (years)	LSEG (Lower Socio Economic Group)		HSEG (Higher Socio Economic Group)	
	Mean Height (cm)	SD	Mean Height (cm)	SD
7	111.84	9.41	117.71	12.68
8	121.57	8.70	128.5	9.01
9	127.35	8.58	133.42	4.20
10	123.52	9.16	138.29	6.90
11	134.89	10.73	138.01	6.95
12	139.35	8.08	136.22	12.00

Table 2. Yearly increment of height according to age groups

Age groups (years)	LSEG (cm) (Height)	HSEG (cm) (Height)
7-8	9.73	10.79
8-9	5.78	4.92
9-10	-3.82	4.87
10-11	11.37	-0.2
11-12	4.46	-1.79

RESULTS

Table 1 shows the description of height based on their age between two socio-economic groups. Table 2 shows yearly increment of height of age groups among two socio-economic groups. In 7-8 age groups of HSEG's yearly increment height (10.79 cm) is higher than LSEG (9.37 cm). On the other hand, in 8-9 age groups LSEG height (5.78 cm) increment is higher than HSEG (4.92 cm). Though height is the most diversified in 10-11 age groups among HSEG (-0.2 cm) rather than LSEG (11.37 cm). For 11-12 age groups, diversity of yearly increment of height score is near among HSEG (4.46 cm) and LSEG (-1.79 cm).

Table 3. Distribution of mid upper arm circumference according to age

Age (years)	LSEG		HSEG	
	Mean MUAC	SD	Mean MUAC	SD
7	15.23	1.90	23.47	6.84
8	18.05	3.51	18.82	3.91
9	17.87	2.61	18.82	3.23
10	16.31	2.51	20.13	3.50
11	21.3	5.55	17.37	2.78
12	20.47	4.21	18.24	3.46

Table 4. Yearly increment of mid upper arm circumference according to age groups

Age groups (years)	LSEG (cm) MUAC	HSEG (cm) MUAC
7-8	2.82	-4.65
8-9	0.18	0
9-10	-1.56	1.31
10-11	4.99	-0.76
11-12	-0.83	0.87

Table 5. Nutritional status of the studied participants based on MUAC

Socio-economic groups	N	Less than equal to 50th percentile (under nutrition)	Greater than equal to 50th percentile (well nourished)
HSEG	81	47 (45%)	41 (54%)
LSEG	104	67 (64.19%)	33 (30.86%)

Table 5 shows the description of mid upper arm (MUAC) circumference based on their age between two socio-economic groups. Table 6 shows yearly increment of MUAC of age groups among two socio-economic groups. We get a picture of increment of MUAC between two socio-economic groups. In HSEG groups, there is a gradual increase of MUAC.

But varied increases and decreases mean rate of MUAC of LSEG. While deviated score is highest at the 7-8 age groups in case of HSEG, the highest deviated score is in 10-11 age groups. In LSEG, 64.19% is under-nutrition and 30.86% is well nourished. In HSEG, 45% is suffered from malnutrition and 54% is well nourished.

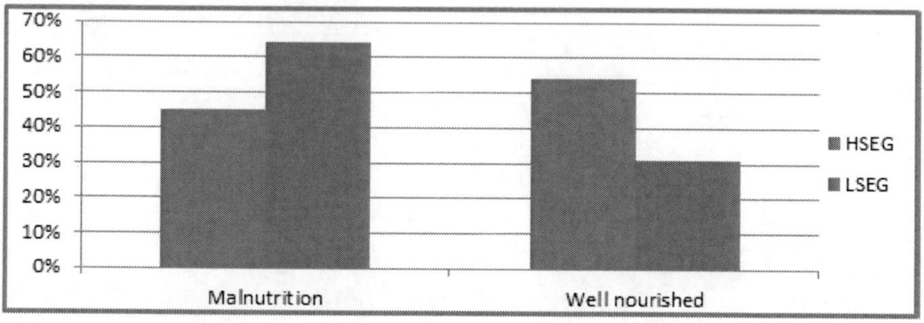

Figure 1. Nutritional status of studied participants based on MUAC.

In HSEG, the stunting participants are 46.91% and wasting participants are 53.08%. In LSEG, stunting participants are 49.03% and wasting participants are 59.61%.

DISCUSSION

There is a significant relationship between parent's knowledge and attitude in the healthy food intake by their children (Srilakshmi, 2019). Overall, there are two significant group and there imbalance in nutrition is clearly deficit in children (Nanclares et al., 2018). In the group of low income there is lack of nutritional practice in participants such as one time rice meal with skipped dinner, with very poor protein intake and less calories. For this imbalance of nutrient there proper growth so more than 80% is in the BMI under-weight category (Ellison, 1982). For the above reason height, MUAC, are very low in this group (Keys, 2015). In the high income group the parents are attracted to the advertisements on television, and buy drinks (Hurlock, 1978). Their diet is also full of first class protein but lack of vitamins and other micronutrients (Snehalatha et al., 2003). The above parameters like MUAC are high and an early sign of overweight is shown in them. The study concludes that both groups of children show nutritional deficiency or imbalance (Nmer et al., 2014). There is a visible incorrect diet and no maintenance in their good health practice by their parents. The income factor was also an important factor seen. Most of the children from lower socio-economic group posses high risk in stunting and wasting. In higher socio-economic group early sign of over weight is noticeable. Lack of parent's idea and knowledge about diet is the main reason behind it. Small sample size was a possible limitation in this study.

Table 6. Distribution of BMI based on age groups

Age groups (years)	HSEG	LSEG
7-8	16.45 ± 4.12 (CED grade II)	16.91 ± 3.60 (CED grade II)
8-9	17.28 ± 4.29 (CED grade I)	17.43 ± 3.45 (CED grade I)
9-10	20.48 ± 5.39 (Normal)	17.45 ± 2.59 (CED grade I)
10-11	20.12 ± 5.44 (Normal)	18.61 ± 3.79 (Normal)
11-12	17.67 ± 4.29 (CED grade I)	19.45 ± 4.21 (Normal)

Table 7. Nutritional status (HAZ and WAZ) of the studied participants

Scio- economic status	N	Stunting	Wasting
HSEG	81	38 (46.91%)	44 (53.08%)
LSEG	104	48 (49.03%)	90 (59.61%)

In addition, parents were not tested with the proper test (Zarnowiecki et al., 2012). This single setting restricts culture and income variations more than if the population had been more diverse; perhaps a mixture of low, middle and high income school. Parent's lack of knowledge regarding nutrition is alarming in healthy food choice and total calorie intake of their children (Ogwu, 2012; Hernandez, 2012). The lack of macro and micro minerals and imbalance in nutrients are visible in the health status of these children (Cameron et al., 1981). To recover this situation, interventions like nutrition camps should be started. That can ensure the enhancement of knowledge in parents about their children's health. Future studies should include responses from a more diverse population. It is advised to question parents regarding their actual knowledge about nutrition (Nanclares et al., 2018).

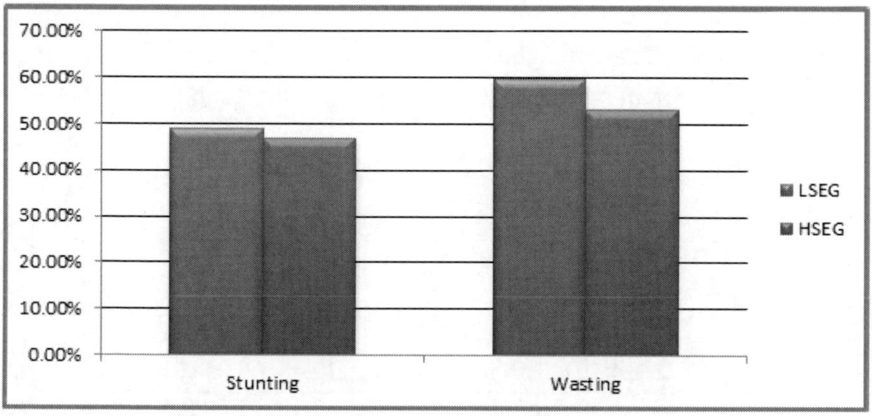

Figure 2. Nutritional status (HAZ and WAZ) of the studied participants.

References

Brug J. 2008. *Determinants of healthy eating: motivation, abilities and environmental opportunities.* https://academic.oup.com/fampra/article/25/suppl_1/i50/542940. Accessed on - 06.08.2019.

Cameron N, Hiemaux J, Jarman S and Tanner JM. 1981. Puberty Rating. *In: LS Lourie (Eds): Practical Human Biology*. London: Academic Press.

Cluss P, Ewing L, King W, Reis E, Dodd J, and Penner B. 2013. *Nutrition knowledge of low-income parents of obese children.* https://www.ncbi.nlm.nih.gov/pmc/articles/PMC3717981/ Accessed on - 06.08.2019.

Elizabeth HB. 1978. Child Growth and Development. *McGraw Hill Education.*

Ellison PT. 1982. Skeletal growth, fatness and menarcheal age: a comparison of two hypotheses. *Human Biology*. 54:269-281.

Fadare O, Amare M, Mavrotas G, Akerele D, Ogunniyi A. 2019. *Mother's nutrition-related knowledge and child nutrition outcomes: Empirical evidence from Nigeria*. https://journals.plos.org/plosone/article?id=10.1371/journal.pone.0212775. Accessed on - 06.08.2019.

Hernandez R. 2012. Parental Knowledge of Poor Dietary Choices Not Enough to Prevent Childhood Obesity, Study Shows. https://www.hopkinsmedicine.org/news/media/releases/parental_knowledge_of_poor_dietary_choices_not_enough_to_prevent_childhood_obesity_study_shows. Accessed on - 06.08.2019.

Keys L. 2015. *The Dietary Habits and Nutrition Education Levels of Parents of Pre-School Children at a Community Head Start Program*. https://pdfs.semanticscholar.org/3a0b/a33e318aec62a3748257acbce5d6b0ab8c7e.pdf. Accessed on - 06.08.2019.

Mc. Nab, Conde F, Mc. Wright, Memish O, Park R, Shaikh S. (Eds). 2016. *Transforming Public Health Surveillance: Proactive Measures for Prevention, Detection, and Response. Elsevier.*

Nanclares A, Zazpe I, Santiago S, Marín L, Campà A, Calvo N. 2018. *Influence of Parental Healthy-Eating Attitudes and Nutritional Knowledge on Nutritional Adequacy and Diet Quality among Preschoolers*: The SENDO Project. https://www.ncbi.nlm.nih.gov/pmc/articles/PMC6316633/. Accessed on - 06.08.2019.

Nirmalan P. 2014. Implications of the Revised Consensus Body Mass Indices for Asian Indians on Clinical Obstetric Practice.*Journal of Clinical and Diagnostic Research.*

Nmer F, Salama A, Elhawary D. 2014. *Nutritional knowledge, attitude, and practice of parents and its impact on growth of their children*. http://mmj.eg.net/article.asp?issn=1110098;year=2014;volume=27;issue=3;spage=612;epage=616;aulast=El-Nmer. Accessed on - 06.08.2019.

Ogwu S. 2012. P*arental Knowledge, Attitudes, and Behaviors about Nutrition and Physical Activity in Relation to BMI of Children with Disability*. Developmental. https://pdfs.semanticscholar.org/4648/98527fb130b5197cca64ee18b52636cd4dbb.pdf. Accessed on - 06.08.2019.

Snehalatha C, Viswanathan V. Ramachandran A. 2003. Cutoff values for normal anthropometric variables in Asian Indian adults. *Diabetes Care*. 26: 1380-1384.

Srilakshmi B. 2019. Dietetics. *New Age International Publisher.*

Tendulkar's survey report, *Report of The Expert Group to Review The Methodology for Estimation of Poverty*. http://planningcommission.nic.in/reports/genrep/rep_pov.pdf. Accessed on - 06.08.2019.

Weiner JS, Lourie JA. 1981. Practical human biology. New York. *Academic Press.*

WHO. 2005. http://www.euro.who.int/en/health-topics/disease-prevention/nutrition/a-healthy-lifestyle/body-mass-index-bmi. Accessed on - 06. 08.2019.

Zarnowiecki D, Sinn N, Petkov J, Dollman J. 2012. *Parental nutrition knowledge and attitudes as predictors of 5-6-year-old children's healthy food.*

In: Contemporary Issues in Childhood … ISBN: 978-1-53617-348-2
Editors: J. Ratan Ghosh and K. Bose ©2020 Nova Science Publishers, Inc.

Chapter 12

MALNUTRITION AND CHILDHOOD INFECTIONS

Jyoti Ratan Ghosh[1,*] and Kaushik Bose[2,†]
[1]Department of Anthropology, Visva-Bharati,
Santiniketan, West Bengal, India
[2]Department of Anthropology,
Vidyasagar University, Midnapore, West Bengal, India

ABSTRACT

Malnutrition refers to deficiencies, excesses, or imbalances in a person's intake of energy and/or nutrients. Malnutrition as a result of disordered nutrient assimilation is also characterized by recurrent infections as well as chronic inflammation, suggesting an underlying immune defect and thus increased susceptibility to infections in children. Infectious disease is one of the primary causes of morbidity and mortality in developing countries, particularly among children. Studies demonstrated impaired immune organ growth, thymic atrophy, preformed T-cell deficiency, altered ratio of T-cell subsets, decreased natural killer (NK) cell

* Corresponding Author's Email: jrghosh@rediffmail.com.
† Corresponding Author's Email: kaushikbose@cantab.net.

activity and cytokine production, decreased T-cell function and the ability of lymphocytes to respond appropriately to cytokines among undernourished infants and children. However, the interrelationship between malnutrition and infections in childhood is complex and much remains to be learned.

Keywords: Malnutrition, undernutrition, infection, immunity, children

INTRODUCTION

Worldwide, 5.6 million children die before their fifth birthday each year, with 80% of these deaths occurring in sub-Saharan Africa and Asia. Almost half of these deaths occur in children with malnutrition (Black et al. 2013). Malnutrition in terms of undernutrition puts children at greater risk of dying from common infections and increases the frequency as well as the severity of such infections, and delays recovery (UNICEF 2019). In 2018, globally there were 149 million children under 5 years of age were stunted, 49 million were wasted and 40 million were overweight (WHO 2019). While known to be a major public health problem in low-income countries, childhood malnutrition is also present in middle-income countries, particularly among marginalized populations (Janevic 2010). Malnutrition among under-five children is also a major public health problem in India, as the prevalence of under-weight children in India is highest in the world, and is nearly double compare to sub-Saharan Africa (Sahu et al. 2015). Nutrition during early infancy and childhood not only affects growth and morbidity in childhood, but also acts as a determinant of nutritional status in adolescent and adult life (Das and Bose 2011). However, in India the problem of malnutrition is a concentrated phenomenon because, a relatively small number of states, districts and villages account for a large share of the malnutrition (Sahu et al. 2015).

The relationship between nutritional status and the immune system has been a topic of study for decades (Shukla et al. 2016). Malnutrition is one of the primary causes of immunodeficiency worldwide, with infants, children, adolescents, and the elderly most affected. There is also a strong association between malnutrition and infection and infant mortality (Katona and Katona-Apte 2008). Several studies have demonstrated that malnutrition impairs host immune responses and is a major cause of secondary immune deficiency (Scrimshaw and SanGiovanni J. P. 1997). Thus, the focus of the present study is to understand the association between malnutrition and infections in children.

MALNUTRITION

Malnutrition refers to deficiencies, excesses, or imbalances in a person's intake of energy and/or nutrients (WHO 2019). The term malnutrition indicates three broad categories namely, undernutrition, which includes wasting (low weight-for-height), stunting (low height-for-age) and underweight (low weight-for-age); micronutrient-related malnutrition, including micronutrient deficiencies (a lack of important vitamins and minerals) or micronutrient excess; and overweight, obesity and diet-related noncommunicable diseases (such as heart disease, stroke, diabetes and some cancers) (WHO 2019).

On the other hand, severe acute malnutrition is commonly categorized into two major syndromes, marasmus and kwashiorkor. Marasmus is defined by a weight-for-height value more than 3 standard deviations below the mean for age and sex (or a weight-for-height z score of less than -3), whereas kwashiorkor is characterized by the presence of bilateral pitting pedal edema, independent of anthropometric values (Grover and Ee 2009). Recently, there has been increased focus on the use of the mid upper arm circumference to understand nutritional status as it is less affected by hydration status and generally it has better predictive value for subsequent mortality than weight-for-height z score (Briend et al. 2016).

Nutritional status can be evaluated in different ways in children including observation and clinical examination, biochemical method and through anthropometric measures (Cross et al. 1995; Das and Bose 2011). However, energy and/or specific nutrient intake, requirements and expenditure are very rarely directly assessed. Instead, practice and research are based on anthropometric measures compared with a reference population (Walson and Berkley 2018). Moreover anthropometric measurements are also inexpensive, non-invasive and suitable for large scale surveys (WHO 1995).

Major factors which modulate nutritional status during early childhood include birth weight, infant and young child feeding practices, morbidity due to infections, treatment of infections, nutrition care during infection and convalescence (Ramachandran and Gopalan 2009). Other established risk factors for malnutrition in low and middle income countries include low household income, while protective factor includes parental education, immunization, and breast feeding (Janevic 2010).

IMMUNE SYSTEM

The immune system was identified as a protective factor during infectious diseases over a century ago (Sattler 2017). The immune system is the body's main defence against foreign materials and biologic agents such as bacteria, viruses, chemicals and foreign cells and tissues (National Research Council 1992). The importance of the immune system to our survival in the face of the wide variety of disease-causing agents is tragically demonstrated by the devastating consequences of the immunological impairment of acquired immune deficiency syndrome and of congenital immunological deficiencies such as severe combined immunodeficiency (SCID) in infants (National Research Council 1989). The immune system can be classified into two subsystems namely, the innate and adaptive immune systems. In general, innate immunity is considered a nonspecific response, whereas the adaptive immune system is thought of as being very specific (Vivier and Malissen 2005).

The combination of these two systems defends the host against infection. Innate immunity provides a first line of protection against pathogens and can be activated rapidly following infection; this response is non-specific and involves epithelial barriers, circulating phagocytes (mainly neutrophils and macrophages), and other cytotoxic cells, such as natural killer cells; further, complement proteins and positive acute-phase proteins (APP) also play an important role (Fearon and Locksley 1996; Medzhitov and Janeway 1998). However, if the infection is not cleared, they activate adaptive immune responses (Greenberg and Grinstein 2002). The function of adaptive immune responses is to destroy invading pathogens and any toxic molecules they produce. Adaptive immune responses are carried out by white blood cells called lymphocytes. There are two broad classes of such responses—antibody responses and cell-mediated immune responses, and they are carried out by different classes of lymphocytes, called B cells and T cells, respectively (Alberts et al. 2002).

MALNUTRITION AND INFECTION

Malnutrition is the failure of the body to get appropriate amounts of nutrients to maintain healthy tissues and organ functions (Oruamabo 2015). Although malnutrition indicates to both states of undernutrition and overnutrition, the present review will emphasise on undernutrition and use the term interchangeably with malnutrition. Malnutrition plays an important role in more than one-third of all child deaths worldwide. Since malnourished children are more susceptible to infections, this combination creates a vicious spiral in which each condition aggravates the other (Page et al. 2013). Malnutrition as a result of disordered nutrient assimilation is also characterized by recurrent infections as well as chronic inflammation, suggesting an underlying immune defect (Olofin et al. 2013; Rytter et al. 2014; Bourke et al. 2016). An infant born with a severely defective immune system will soon die unless appropriate measures are taken to isolate it from a host of infectious agents, including bacteria, viruses, fungi and parasites (Alberts et al. 2002). It is well documented that the development of infant immunity during the first two and half years of life is very sensitive to nutritional status (Bourke et al. 2016). Number of studies demonstrated impaired immune organ growth, thymic atrophy, preformed T-cell deficiency, altered ratio of T-cell subsets, decreased natural killer (NK) cell activity and cytokine production, decreased T-cell function and the ability of lymphocytes to respond appropriately to cytokines among undernourished infants and children (Prentice 1999; Rodriguez et al. 2011; Prentice et al. 2013; Moore et al. 2014; Rytter et al. 2014). However, the host defence mechanisms depend upon the activities of white blood cells to function. In severely malnourished children these defence mechanisms, including both acquired (lymphocyte functions) and innate (macrophages and granulocytes) are affected. As a result, malnourished children with weak immunity become more susceptible to infections (Schaible and Kaufmann 2007; Rodriguez et al. 2011). Moreover, frequent infections in children are also associated with lower growth velocity and stunting (Checkley et al. 2008; Guerrant et al. 2008; Rodrıguez et al. 2011). Infection and the presence of higher inflammation are also associated with growth suppression as both of these are linked to growth hormone resistance (DeBoer et al. 2017).

In order to efficiently fight against infections, innate protective mechanisms of the body such as intact skin surface and naso-oesopharyngeal linings, gastrointestinal, genito-urinary tracts as well as capability to produce mucous secretions are necessary to provide a barrier to invasion (Rodriguez et al. 2011; Shukla et al. 2016). However, in order to do this a range of nutrients including antioxidant enzymes, minerals and vitamin are needed by the body (Calder and Jackson 2000). This might be the reason that malnourished children are commonly characterise by varying degrees of mucous membrane disruptions and abnormalities in protective secretions along with nutrient deficiencies, which make them prone to infections (Rodriguez et al. 2011; Shukla et al. 2016; Chiabi et al. 2018).

Defects in adaptive immune function include reduced levels of soluble IgA in saliva and tears, lymphoid organ atrophy, delayed-type hypersensitivity responses, fewer circulating B cells, a shift from Th1-associated to Th2-associated cytokines, and lymphocyte hyporesponsiveness to phytohemagglutinin, but preserved lymphocyte and immunoglobulin levels in peripheral blood (Rytter et al. 2014). The availability of complement components and phagocyte function are also compromised due to malnutrition, which in turns directly affects the pathogen elimination process (Chandra 2002; França et al. 2009). A number of studies demonstrated that the biological function of different cell types (B lymphocytes, macrophages and Kupffer cells) is clearly decreased during nutritional deficiencies (Redmond et al. 1991; Petro et al. 1994; Honda et al., 1995; Stapleton et al. 2001; França et al. 2009). Atrophy in the primary lymphoid organs due to malnutrition in new-borns and infants also affect the production of B and T cell repertoires (França et al. 2009). Moreover, malnutrition in new-borns and small children also provokes thymus atrophy that, in turn, reduces thymus cell number and also severely affects the development of peripheral lymphoid organs (Savino 2002). Several studies have demonstrated that protein-calorie malnutrition also impairs cell-mediated immunity (Scrimshaw and SanGiovanni 1997).

Though malnutrition makes children susceptible to infections, infectious could also results in undernutrition among children. Study demonstrated that gastrointestinal infection can cause prolonged diarrhoea leading to loss of nutrients and malnutrition (Pelletier et al. 1993; Schaible and Kaufmann 2007; Shukla et al. 2016). Moreover, acquired immune deficiency syndrome, tuberculosis and intestinal parasites along with other chronic infections may also cause cachexia and anaemia (Schaible and Kaufmann 2007). In conclusion, the interrelationship between malnutrition and infections in childhood is complex and much remains to be learned. However, there is a serious need for studies to generate knowledge for better understanding this interrelationship to reduce childhood malnutrition.

REFERENCES

Alberts, B., Johnson, A., Lewis, J., Raff, M., Roberts, K., Walter, P. 2002. *Molecular biology of the cell.* New York: Garland Science.

Black, R. E., Victora, C. G., Walker, S. P., Bhutta, Z. A., Christian, P., de Onis, M., Ezzati, M., Grantham-McGregor, S., Katz, J., Martorell, R., Uauy, R. Maternal and Child Nutrition Study Group. Maternal and child nutrition study group. 2013. Gaternal and child undernutrition and overweight in low-income and middle-income countries. *Lancet,* 2013; 382:427 - 451.

Bourke, C. D., Berkley, J. A., Prendergast, A. J. 2016. Immune dysfunction as a cause and consequence of malnutrition. *Trends in Immunology,* 37: 386-398.

Briend, A., Alvarez, J. L., Avril, N.,Bahwere, P., Bailey, J., Berkley, J. A., Binns, P., Blackwell, N., Dale, N., Deconinck, H., Delchevalerie, P., Dent, N., Gallagher, M., Guerrero, S., Hanson, K., Kerac, M., Manary, M., Mwangome, M. K., Myatt, M., Phelan, K. P. Q., Pietzsch, S., Ubach, N. S.,Shepherd, S., Kam, S. V. D., Vargas, A., Whitney, S. 2016. Low mid-upper arm circumference identifies children with a high risk of death who should be the priority target for treatment. *BMC Nutrition,* 2:63.

Calder, P. C., Jackson, A. A. 2000. Undernutrition, infection and immune function. *Nutrition Research Reviews*, 13:3-29.

Chandra, R. K. 2002. Nutrition and the immune system from birth to old age. *European Journal of Clinican Nutrition,* 56:S73-6.

Checkley, W., Buckley, G., Gilman, R. H., Assis, A. M., Guerrant, R. L., Morris, S. S., Mølbak, K., Valentiner-Branth, P., Lanata, C. F., Black, R. E. Childhood Malnutrition and Infection Network. 2008. Multi-country analysis of the effects of diarrhoea on childhood stunting. *International Journal of Epidemiology,* 37:816 - 30.

Chiabi, A., Obadeyi, B., Nguefack, F. D., Chiabi, R. M., Berinyuy, E. N.,Chiabi, E. N., Mbang, T. A., Obama, M. T.2018.The vicious cycle of malnutrition and childhood infections – what are the policy implications?*Archives of Pediatrics and Neonatology*, 1:21-25.

Cross, J. H., Holden, C., MacDonald, A., Pearmain, G., Stevens, M. C. G., Booth, I. W. 1995. Clinical examination compared with anthropometry in evaluating nutritional status. *Archives of Disease in Childhood,* 72:60-61.

Das, S., Bose, K. 2011. Prevalence of thinness among Santal preschool children using new body mass index cut-off points. *Journal of Anthropology*, 2011: 602782.

DeBoer, M. D., Scharf, R. J., Leite, A. M., Ferrer, A., Havt, A., Pinkerton, R., Lima, A. A., Guerrant, R. L. 2017. Systemic inflammation, growth factors, and linear growth in the setting of infection and malnutrition. *Nutrition,* 33: 248 - 253.

Fearon, D. T., Locksley, R. M. 1996. The instructive role of innate immunity in the acquired immune response. *Science,*272: 50-54.

França, T. G. D., Ishikawa, L. L. W., Zorzella-Pezavento, S. F. G., Chiuso-Minicucci, F., da Cunha, M. L. R. S., Sartori, A. 2009. Impact of malnutrition on immunity and infection. *Journal of Venomous Animals and Toxins including Tropical Diseases*, 15:374-390.

Greenberg, S., Grinstein, S. 2002. Phagocytosis and innate immunity. *Current Opinion in Immunology,*14: 136-145.

Grover, Z., Ee, L. C. 2009. Protein energy malnutrition. *Pediatric Clinics of North America,* 56:1055 - 1068.

Guerrant, R. L., Oria, R. B., Moore, S. R., Oria, M. O., Lima, A. A. 2008. Malnutrition as an enteric infectious disease with long-term effects on child development. *Nutrition Reviews*, 66:487 - 505.

Honda, M., Kamiyama, Y., Kawamura, K., Kawahara, K., Shishido, S., Nakai, H., Kawamura, T., Ito, H. 1995. Growth, development and nutritional status in Japanese children under 2 years on continuous ambulatory peritoneal dialysis. *Pediatric Nephrology,* 9:543-8.

Janevic, T., Petrovic, O., Bjelic, I., Kubera, A. 2010. Risk factors for childhood malnutrition in Roma settlements in Serbia. *BMC Public Health,*10:509.

Katona, P., Katona-Apte, J. 2008. The interaction between nutrition and infection. *Clinical Infectious Diseases*, 46:1582 - 1588.

Medzhitov, R., Janeway, C. A. Jr. 1998. An ancient system of host defense. *Current Opinion in Immunology,*10: 12-15.

Moore, S. E. Fulford, A. J. C., Wagatsuma, Y., Persson, L. A., Arifeen, S. E., Prentice, A. M. 2014. Thymus development and infant and child mortality in rural Bangladesh. *International Journal of Epidemiology,* 43, 216 - 223.

National Research Council. 1989. *Opportunities in Biology.* Washington, DC: The National Academies Press.

National Research Council. 1992. *Biologic Markers in Immunotoxicology.* Washington, DC: The National Academies Press.

Olofin, I., McDonald, C. M., Ezzati, M., Flaxman, S., Black, R. E., Fawzi, W. W., Caulfield, L. E., Danaei, G. 2013. Associations of suboptimal growth with all-cause and cause-specific mortality in children under five years: a pooled analysis of ten prospective studies. *PLoS ONE,* 8: e64636.

Oruamabo, R. S. 2015. Child malnutrition and the Millennium Development Goals: much haste but less speed. *Archives of Disease in Childhood,* 100: s19-22.

Page, A. L., de Rekeneire, N., Sayadi, S., Aberrane, S., Janssens, A. C., Rieux, C., Djibo, A., Manuguerra, J. C., Ducou-le-Pointe, H., Grais, R. F., Schaefer, M., Guerin, P. J., Baron, E. 2013. Infections in children admitted with complicated severe acute malnutrition in Niger. *PLoS ONE,* 8: e68699.

Pelletier, D., Frongillo, E., Habicht, J. P. 1993. Epidemiologic evidence for a potentiating effect of malnutrition on child mortality. *American Journal of Public Health,*83: 1130-1133.

Petro, T. M., Schwartz, K. M., Chen, S. S. A. 1994. Production of IL2 and IL3 in syngeneic mixed lymphocyte reactions of BALB/c mice are elevated during a period of moderate dietary protein deficiency. *Immunological Investigations,* 23:143-52.

Prentice, A. M., Ward, K. A., Goldberg, G. R., Jarjou, L. M., Moore, S. E., Fulford, A. J., Prentice, A. 2013. Critical windows for nutritional interventions against stunting. *American Journal of Clinical Nutrition,* 97: 911 - 918.

Prentice, A. M. 1999. The thymus: a barometer of malnutrition. *British Journal of Nutrition,* 81: 345 - 347.

Ramachandran, P., Gopalan, H. S. 2009. Undernutrition and risk of infections in preschool children. *Indian Journal of Medical Research,* 130: 579-583.

Redmond, H. P., Shou, J., Kelly, C. J., Schreiber, S., Miller, E., Leon, P., Daly, J. M. 1991. Immunosuppressive mechanisms in protein-calorie malnutrition. *Surgery*, 110:311-7.

Rytter, M. J., Kolte, L., Briend, A., Friis, H., Christensen, V. B. 2014. The immune system in children with malnutrition–a systematic review. *PLoS ONE*, 9: e105017.

Sahu, S. K., Kumar, S. G., Bhat, B. V., Premarajan, K. C., Sarkar, S., Roy, G., Joseph, N. 2015. Malnutrition among under-five children in India and strategies for control. *Journal of Natural Science, Biology and Medicine,*6: 18 - 23.

Sattler, S. 2017. The role of the immune system beyond the fight against infection. *Advances in Experimental Medicine and Biology,* 1003:3-14.

Savino, W. 2002. The thymus gland is a target in malnutrition. *European Journal of Clinican Nutrition,* 56:S46-9.

Schaible, U. E., Kaufmann, S. H. E. 2007. Malnutrition and infection: Complex mechanisms and global impacts. *PLoS Med.,* 4: e115.

Scrimshaw, N. S., SanGiovanni, J. P. 1997. Synergism of nutrition, infection, and immunity: an overview. *American Journal of Clinical Nutrition,* 66: 464S-477S.

Shukla, Y., Verma, P., Tiwari, R., Kasar, P. K., Tomar, S. P. 2016. Association of severe acute malnutrition with infections in under-five children admitted to Nutritional Rehabilitation Center—study from central India. *International Journal of Medical Science and Public Health,* 5: 758-763.

Stapleton, P. P., Fujita, J., Murphy, E. M., Naama, H. A., Daly, J. M. 2001. The influence of restricted calorie intake on peritoneal macrophage function. *Nutrition,* 17:41-5.

Vivier, E., Malissen, B. 2005. Innate and adaptive immunity: specificities and signaling hierarchies revisited. *Nature Immunology,* 6:17-21.

Walson, J. L., Berkley, J. A. 2018. The impact of malnutrition on childhood infections. *Current Opinion in Infectious Diseases*, 31:231 - 236.

World Health Organization (WHO). 2019. *Child malnutrition.* https://www.who.int/gho/child-malnutrition/en/ accessed on 28.07. 2019.

World Health Organization (WHO). 2019. *Malnutrition.* https://www.who.int/topics/malnutrition/en/, accessed on 21.07.2019.

World Health Organization. 1995. *Physical status: the use and interpretation of anthropometry.* Technical Report Series no. 854. World Health Organization, Geneva.

About the Editors

Jyoti Ratan Ghosh, PhD
Assistant Professor
Department of Anthropology
Visva-Bharati University
Santiniketan, West Bengal, India
Email: jrghosh@rediffmail.com

Dr. Jyoti Ratan Ghosh is an Assistant Professor at the Department of Anthropology, Visva-Bharati University, Santiniketan, West Bengal, India. Dr. Ghosh obtained his B.Sc. (Hons.) Degree in Anthropology in 2001 and M.Sc. Degree in Anthropology in 2003 from the University of Calcutta. He was awarded Ph.D. in Anthropology by the University of Calcutta in 2008.

Dr. Ghosh was awarded Gansu International Fellowship in China by the *People's Republic of China in 2018.* His research is focused on human growth and body composition, human nutrition, forensic anthropology and non-communicable diseases. He has in his credit research project of University Grants Commission as well as more than sixty research papers in national, international journals and books.

Kaushik Bose, PhD, DSc

Professor
Department of Anthropology
Vidyasagar University
Midnapore, West Bengal, India
Email: kaushikbose@cantab.net

Dr. Kaushik Bose is a Professor at the Department of Anthropology, Vidyasagar University, India. He has been the recipient of several scholarships, fellowships and medals. He is a Member/Fellow of several professional bodies including Unit for the Biocultural Variation and Obesity, Oxford University. He was the recipient of a Commonwealth Scholarship and obtained his Ph.D. from Cambridge University in 1996.He was at Queens' College, Cambridge. Earlier he had obtained his PhD degree from Panjab University, India. He also worked as a Post-Doctoral Fellow at the Department of Nutrition and Dietetics, King's College London. He was awarded a D.Sc. degree by Vidyasagar University in 2016.

He has published more than 260 research papers besides editing seven books. He is the editor of the Journal of Life Sciences. His research interests are anthropometry and body composition; particularly ethnic variation in health and disease.

He has undertaken collaborative research with several institutes including USAID, Tufts University, FHI360 (Washington, D.C.) and Polish Academy of Sciences, Wroclaw.

LIST OF CONTRIBUTORS

Aditi Bardhan
Sociological Research Unit, Indian Statistical Institute, 203 BT Road, Kolkata 700108, India

Premananda Bharati
Professor (Retd.), Biological Anthropology Unit, Indian Statistical Institute, 203 BT Road, Kolkata 700108, India

Susmita Bharati
Professor, Sociological Research Unit, Indian Statistical Institute, 203 BT Road, Kolkata 700108, India

Barry Bogin
Professor,Loughborough University, School of Sport, Exercise & Health Sciences, LE113TU, UK

Diptendu Chatterjee
Assistant Professor, Department of Anthropology, University of Calcutta

Priyanka Dhara
Research Student, Department of Anthropology, Visva-Bharati University, Bolpur, Birbhum, WB, India

Dali Dutta
Department of Anthropology, Dibrugarh University, Dibrugarh

Rima Ghosh
Research Student, Department of Nutrition, Vidyasagar University

Helmizar
Department of Nutrition, Faculty of Public Health, Andalas University, Padang, Indonesia

Michael Hermanussen
Professor, Aschauhof, 24340Eckernförde - Altenhof, Germany

Md. Golam Hossain
Professor, Health Research Group, Department of Statistics, University of Rajshahi, Rajshahi-6205, Bangladesh

Md. Reazul Karim
Health Research Group, Department of Statistics, University of Rajshahi, Rajshahi-6205, Bangladesh

Pikli Khanra
Research Student, Department of Anthropology, Vidyasagar University, Midnapore – 721 102, West Bengal, India

NurIndrawaty Lipoeto
Department of Nutrition, Faculty of Medicine, Andalas University, Padang, Indonesia

Dilip Mahalanabis
Society for Applied studies, CF-198, Salt Lake City, Sector 1, Kolkata – 700 064, India

M Siva Durga Prasad Nayak
Assistant professor, Department of Community Medicine, RIMS Medical College/ NTRHUS, India

Manoranjan Pal
Economic Research Unit, Indian Statistical Institute, 203 BT Road, Kolkata 700108, India

Paulina Pruszkowska-Przybylska
Department of Anthropology, Faculty of Biology and Environmental Protection, University of Łódź, 90-237, Poland

Masud Rana
Health Research Group, Department of Statistics, University of Rajshahi, Rajshahi-6205, Bangladesh

Shreyasi Roy
UGC-NET Junior Research Fellow, Department of Anthropology, University of North Bengal, NBU Campus, Raja Rammohunpur, Darjeeling-734 013, West Bengal, India

Christiane Scheffler
University of Potsdam, Institute of Biochemistry and Biology, Human Biology, Maulbeerallee 2a, 14469 Potsdam, Germany

Bandana Sen
Society for Applied studies, CF-198, Salt Lake City, Sector 1, Kolkata – 700 064, India

Jaydip Sen
Professor, Department of Anthropology, University of North Bengal, NBU Campus, Raja Rammohunpur, Darjeeling-734 013, West Bengal, India

Sarthak Sengupta
Professor, Department of Anthropology, Dibrugarh University, Dibrugarh

Sunita Sreegiri
Associate professor, Department of Community Medicine, Andhra Medical College/ NTRHUS, India

Abdul Wadood
Deputy Chief Medical Officer, University of Rajshahi, Rajshahi, Bangladesh

INDEX

B

C

F

G

H

U

W